Using CBT in General Practice

2nd Edition

The 10 Minute CBT Handbook

Lee David

MBBS, BSc, MRCGP, MA in cognitive behavioural therapy
GP and Cognitive Behavioural Therapist, Hertfordshire

Scion

© Scion Publishing Ltd, 2013

ISBN 978 1 904842 93 4

Second edition first published in 2013

First edition published 2006, reprinted 2009, 2010, 2011, 2012, 2013

A CIP catalogue record for this book is available from the British Library.

Scion Publishing Limited
The Old Hayloft, Vantage Business Park, Bloxham Road, Banbury, Oxfordshire OX16 9UX, UK
www.scionpublishing.com

Important Note from the Publisher
The information contained within this book was obtained by Scion Publishing Limited from sources believed by us to be reliable. However, while every effort has been made to ensure its accuracy, no responsibility for loss or injury whatsoever occasioned to any person acting or refraining from action as a result of information contained herein can be accepted by the authors or publishers.

Although every effort has been made to ensure that all owners of copyright material have been acknowledged in this publication, we would be pleased to acknowledge in subsequent reprints or editions any omissions brought to our attention.

Readers should remember that medicine is a constantly evolving science and while the authors and publishers have ensured that all dosages, applications and practices are based on current indications, there may be specific practices which differ between communities. You should always follow the guidelines laid down by the manufacturers of specific products and the relevant authorities in the country in which you are practising.

Typeset by Phoenix Photosetting, Chatham, Kent, UK
Printed by Charlesworth Press, Wakefield, UK

Contents

Preface

Using CBT in General Practice aims to be a practical handbook, which contains a comprehensive overview of CBT principles and their application within primary care. It was written with the needs of busy GPs in mind. It reviews the basic principles of cognitive-behavioural therapy (CBT) and techniques for applying these within brief consultations. The book also provides an overview of many common primary care problems that can benefit from a CBT approach, including emotional disorders and psychological difficulties associated with chronic physical disease.

This book is aimed at GPs and other health professionals who have a role in promoting the emotional wellbeing of patients, including nurses, health visitors, occupational therapists, physios, speech therapists, and counsellors. For the sake of simplicity, I have used the term 'GP' throughout the book.

As a GP myself, I fully appreciate the enormous challenges and pressures of working in primary care. During my postgraduate training in CBT, I was struck by how valuable the training was to my practice as a GP. I also discovered that I *already* possessed many of the skills required for effective CBT, and this is also true for most health professionals that I work with. I now find that CBT strategies have become part of my daily repertoire of communication skills that I use routinely within consultations.

10 Minute CBT offers an innovative approach to teaching CBT to primary care health professionals, which was designed to be used within the 'real-life' setting of primary care. The feedback from our workshops and training events has shown that simple perspectives and concepts from CBT are effective and useful within routine GP appointments, and have significant benefits for both patient and health professional.

Lee David
May 2013

Introduction

How to use this book

Using CBT in General Practice is divided into three sections.
- Section A is an introduction to the theory and application of cognitive-behavioural approaches in the primary care setting.
- Section B introduces some more advanced techniques and theory of CBT.
- Section C is a clinical reference section. Each chapter provides an overview of a common psychological disorder and describes a cognitive behavioural approach to helping patients with the problem.

It is important for readers to learn and develop their skills and understanding of CBT, not simply by reading this book, but through *practice*. To facilitate this 'hands-on' learning, a variety of practical exercises have been included in most chapters. These will help readers to incorporate CBT theory into their own practice.

About the author

I am a part-time GP Partner and Trainer based in St Albans, Hertfordshire. I have a Masters in counselling (cognitive-behavioural) and also practice as a CBT therapist. I am director of the organisation 10 Minute CBT, which provides CBT training workshops for GPs and other health professionals throughout the UK and internationally.

Lee David
MB BS, BSc, MRCGP, MA in CBT
Director of 10 Minute CBT
GP and CBT therapist
www.10MinuteCBT.co.uk

Acknowledgements

I would like to express my gratitude to the many people who have encouraged and supported me in writing this book. I would also like to thank all the CBT trainers and the admin team at 10 Minute CBT for their hard work and dedication. I am very grateful to Scion Publishing, especially my editor,

Jonathan Ray, for his patience and continued encouragement to help me complete this second edition.

My greatest appreciation and love must go to my family: Fran, Elissa and Miles, who are the most important part of my life by far, and who give meaning to everything that I do. And thank you to my parents, Cat and George, whose endless support and love have encouraged me throughout my life.

Chapter 1

Introduction to CBT

What is CBT?

Cognitive-behavioural therapy (CBT) is a structured psychological therapy which helps people to understand and overcome a wide range of emotional and physical difficulties. CBT views problems as arising from interactions between cognitions (thoughts), emotion, behaviour and physiological processes. It takes a problem-focused, skills-based approach which aims to improve distressing physical and emotional symptoms, re-evaluate unhelpful thoughts and encourage helpful behavioural reactions.

The term CBT encompasses a wide range of treatment approaches, including one-to-one therapy, group therapy, and supported or individual use of self-help materials. CBT can be used alone or in combination with medication, depending on the severity or nature of the individual patient's problem. It is also important to note that CBT can be used effectively with a wide range of patient groups, irrespective of ability, culture, race, gender or sexual preference.

Key aspects of a CBT approach include the following:
- Patients and therapists work in a collaborative partnership to jointly identify, understand and overcome the patient's difficulties.
- Structured and problem-focused; it involves setting specific goals and monitoring outcomes.
- Empowering for patients who develop lasting practical skills in understanding and managing their own problems.
- Time-limited and brief (usually 6–20 sessions), depending on the particular problem and severity.
- Takes a 'here and now' approach to targeting distressing symptoms rather than 'root causes', childhood or past problems.
- Uses a questioning style known as guided discovery to identify each patient's unique viewpoint and beliefs, and to stimulate recognition of alternative, more helpful perspectives and ideas.
- Uses behavioural experiments to test the accuracy of alternative beliefs, enabling patients to learn new ways of thinking and acting.
- Uses 'homework' to set tasks for the patient to try out between therapy sessions, putting what has been learned into practice.

Why is CBT important in primary care?

The vast majority of mental health problems are managed within the primary care setting; as many as 25% of GP consultations are for patients with mental disorders and these patients consult GPs around twice as often as other patients (DoH, 2001). In general practice, 10–15% of patients are suffering from major depression and as many as two to three times more are experiencing depressive symptoms which do not meet diagnostic criteria for major depressive disorder (Katon & Schulberg, 1992).

CBT has been shown to be an effective treatment for a wide variety of common mental health problems (DoH, 2001; NICE, 2008, 2009a & 2009b), including:
- depression
- panic disorder
- generalised anxiety disorder
- phobias (including social phobia and agoraphobia)
- obsessive–compulsive disorder
- health anxiety, medically unexplained symptoms and somatisation disorder (Escobar *et al.*, 2007, Speckens *et al.*, 1995, Warwick *et al.*, 1996)
- post-traumatic stress disorder (PTSD)
- eating disorders (including anorexia and bulimia).

The National Institute for Health and Clinical Excellence (NICE, 2009a & 2011) have highlighted CBT as the first-line psychological therapy for the management of both depression and anxiety. There is also growing evidence that CBT is an effective approach to improving physical and emotional outcomes in a range of common chronic physical diseases, including diabetes, chronic airway disease, cardiovascular disease, chronic pain, and bowel disorders (DoH, 2008; Waddell *et al.*, 2008).

Access to CBT

Increasing investment in training CBT therapists in the *Improving Access to Psychological Therapies* (IAPT) programme is likely to shorten waiting lists for CBT. The potential benefits of improved access to CBT include (NICE, 2008):
- improved symptoms (or reduced risk of deterioration)
- reduced suicide risk
- reducing prescriptions for antidepressant medications
- reduced referrals to secondary care services
- benefits in the workplace – reduced sick leave and better retention in employment
- improved quality of patient-centred clinical care through increasing patient choice, experience and engagement.

What is '10 Minute CBT'?

10 Minute CBT is an approach to bringing CBT principles in 'bite-sized' chunks into brief consultations within the routine practice of busy health professionals, rather than within specialist clinics. It can be used as an alternative, or in addition to, other strategies, including medication, use of self-help materials and referral for formal therapy.

10 Minute CBT includes realistic, practical skills which build on a GP's existing repertoire of communication skills and mental health expertise – a new 'tool' to add to the GP 'toolkit'.

There are many benefits to using a 10 Minute CBT approach for both health professionals and patients (*Box 1.1*).

Box 1.1

Benefits from applying brief CBT skills within primary care

Benefits for health professionals

- Increased confidence and skill in diagnosis and management of common psychological and emotional disorders
- Personal and job satisfaction – consultations are more interesting and enjoyable
- Improved time management – more effective use of time
- Able to use effective cognitive and behavioural strategies for facilitating change
- Helps understand and improve relationships with patients, including 'heartsink' patients
- Useful for coping with GPs' own difficulties and problems
- Also useful for teaching, mentoring and clinical supervision

Benefits for patients

- Improved relationships with health professionals – increased empathy and shared understanding of difficulties helps patients feel better understood and listened to
- Improved ability to understand and make sense of their problems
- Aids discovery of new coping strategies or solutions to problems
- Reduction in distressing emotional symptoms
- Better able to manage physical and emotional health (improved self-efficacy skills)

The main aim of 10 Minute CBT is to promote patient empowerment and facilitate self-help skills for patients, rather than necessarily being responsible for providing a 'cure' for the patient's problems. The main roles for the GP include:

- engaging the patient's interest in the potential for change
- increasing patient understanding and insight into their problems
- supporting the ability of patients to identify new perspectives and coping strategies for managing their problems *themselves.*

The cognitive-behavioural model (CBM) (*Figure 1.1*) provides a focused and simple five areas framework for incorporating CBT into a brief consultation. The health professional can help the patient map out their problems according to this structured model, and ask questions that encourage the patient to reflect and learn from the discussion. This will be discussed in more detail in *Chapter 3.*

Other 10 Minute CBT skills suitable for brief consultations include focusing on effective behavioural change strategies, such as behavioural activation and goal setting; these are easier to apply in brief consultations than many cognitive techniques.

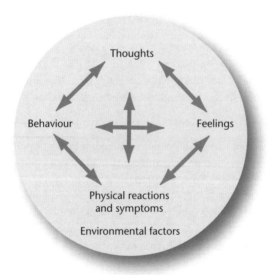

Figure 1.1:   Cognitive-behavioural model (CBM) for GP consultations (adapted from Padesky & Mooney, 1990; Williams & Garland, 2002)

Case Example 1.1: How GPs are using 10 Minute CBT

"A patient experienced panic attacks for a few years… basically we tried to explore how he was responding to a panic attack, what his reaction to it was and whether there was any trigger that he was unaware of. We managed to find out that there was a relationship between things happening at work and the panic attacks and also the way he was actually dealing with them was probably causing [more] anxiety. And he did manage to decrease the number of panic attacks and also to lift, to experience the panic attacks in a much less distracting way. And he was really pleased, in fact he said he didn't go to therapy afterwards because he felt he was able to… his words were, 'You know, you helped me and now I feel I can deal with that.' So that was quite nice."
GP, London

"I had a lady coming for about five or six months with chest pain. She's under cardiologists privately, had all the investigations and there's no cardiac or respiratory cause found. We think it's probably all anxiety-related. I have seen her so many times and the minute she feels slightly unwell, she rings straight away and thinks she's got a serious heart problem. So we worked on how this is sort of a vicious cycle and that if she comes in and we reassure her it's reinforcing her behaviour. We try to address some of the triggers that could be causing that. It's definitely had an impact. I still think she does have this underlying anxiety and we haven't got rid of it completely. But I think, yeah, I definitely think that she's improving."
GP, London

Basic principles of CBT

The fundamental principle of CBT is that the way people *think* in a specific situation will affect how they *feel* emotionally and physically, and will also alter their *behaviour* (and vice versa).

Depressed and anxious people often adopt extreme, unhelpful and negative thinking patterns, viewing themselves as worthless, a failure or vulnerable to danger. These negative beliefs lead to a change in their behaviour, perhaps reducing social activities, avoiding anxiety-provoking situations, or unhelpful new behaviours such as excessive drinking or self-harm. These behavioural changes create a 'vicious cycle' of increasing emotional distress.

Different perspectives for the same situation

One of the first steps in CBT is to separate people's internal reactions from the external situations that have triggered the response. People often blame a difficult event or situation for their emotional reactions:

Event	→	Emotion
I failed my exam	→	I feel depressed

Yet many different individuals react very differently to similar situations or events. Some people cope well with even major life events such as a bereavement or serious illness, whilst others become highly anxious or depressed when faced with common difficulties and pressures. From this observation arises the very important CBT principle, that it is not the event itself which leads to feelings and behaviour, but the thoughts and beliefs which give meaning to the event for a particular individual.

Event	→	Thought	→	Emotion
I failed my exam	→	I'm useless and I'll never get a job	→	I feel depressed

Box 1.2	The tale of the Chinese farmer

The tale of the Chinese farmer

There is an old Chinese tale about a farmer whose horse ran away.

"What terrible luck," said his neighbour.

"Good luck, bad luck. Nobody knows for sure," said the farmer.

A few days later, the horse returned, bringing with it five more beautiful horses from the wild.

"What fantastic luck," said the neighbour.

"Good luck, bad luck. Nobody knows for sure," said the farmer.

The next day, the farmer's son fell and broke his leg when trying to break in the new horses.

"What bad luck," said the neighbour.

"Good luck, bad luck. Nobody knows for sure," said the farmer.

The next week, the army came to the area, looking to recruit all young men to the armed forces. They came to the farm, but because the farmer's son had a broken leg, they passed by and he was allowed to remain with his father.

"What good luck," said the neighbour.

"Good luck, bad luck. Nobody knows for sure," said the farmer.

This is illustrated further in the following situation:

You have cooked dinner for a friend, who is usually very reliable. An hour after she was due to arrive, there is still no sign and you have received no phone call...

How would you react in this situation? The following table illustrates four possible different reactions, broken down into thoughts with their corresponding feelings and behaviours:

Event	A friend is an hour late for dinner...			
Thought	*How dare she do this to me! She is so inconsiderate and rude!*	*She probably didn't want to come because she doesn't really like me. I'm such a loser.*	*What if she's had an accident? She could be seriously hurt.*	*I expect she's stuck in traffic. At least I have extra time to prepare dinner.*
Feelings	Anger	Depression	Anxiety	Relieved
Physical reactions	Tension in neck and arms	Fatigue	Racing heart, sweating	Nothing in particular
Possible behaviour	Tell her off or act unfriendly when she arrives	Withdraw from people and stop asking them over	Phone local hospitals	Continue preparing dinner

Of course, any one of these responses may be appropriate in different circumstances, but persistently negative thinking styles can lead to emotional disorders such as depression or anxiety disorders.

From *theory* to *practice*...	Start becoming aware of the diverse range of reactions both in yourself and others to different situations in everyday life. Take particular note of the following: • Are there any links between people's thoughts, feelings and how they behave? • What is the impact of this behaviour? How is it helpful or unhelpful?

Key learning points

- CBT is an effective, evidence-based treatment for many emotional and physical health disorders that are very common and form a significant proportion of the primary care workload.
- GPs *already* possess many of the skills required to learn and use CBT in their consultations.
- In CBT it is the interpretation of an event, rather than the event, which is viewed as causing emotional distress.
- Negative thoughts, feelings, physical symptoms and behaviour often link to form 'vicious cycles' which maintain problems and emotional distress.
- Using a five areas or cognitive-behavioural model as a framework helps patients make sense of their problems and may identify new strategies for breaking vicious cycles and making change.
- The main role of a 10 Minute CBT approach in general practice is to help the patient understand and find ways to overcome problems for themselves.

Chapter 2

Adapting CBT for general practice

Practical aspects of incorporating CBT into brief consultations

10 Minute CBT can be used flexibly by health professionals in a variety of different practices and patient populations. Simple CBT-based communication skills can be used on an ad hoc basis in any consultation. These include identifying and reflecting back a patient's key thoughts, feelings and behaviour, using empowering CBT-based explanations of problems, or gently encouraging positive behavioural change.

It can also be helpful to plan a specific appointment to explore problems in more detail using a brief CBT approach. Ideally, try to agree this in advance, giving the patient time to think about their problems before the consultation. Many GPs plan a slightly longer appointment (e.g. 20 minutes) at times when they are less busy or feel less pressured, such as at the start or end of a surgery. This may act as an investment of time, which reduces repeat attendances and may save time in the long term.

Continuity is also helpful, and you could offer one or more review sessions over a period of time. There is no set rule about how many appointments should be offered in this way, with the number usually depending on available time.

Choice of patients

10 Minute CBT can be used for a wide range of emotional and physical conditions. Suitable patients include those who do not wish to attend 'formal' therapy, as well as those on waiting lists or those experiencing relapses of symptoms following standard CBT interventions.

The approach is particularly helpful for patients with mild to moderate emotional problems and also to help understand psychological aspects of physical illness. Relevant conditions include:
- depression
- anxiety, worry and panic attacks
- chronic pain
- psychological elements of physical disease

- promoting healthy lifestyles and behaviours (e.g. encouraging weight loss, exercise or smoking cessation)
- health anxiety and medically unexplained symptoms.

Patients who are particularly likely to benefit from CBT include those who understand and relate to the CBT model, and who are motivated to engage with a psychological approach (see *Box 2.1*).

Box 2.1

Features suggesting that patients are likely to be suitable for CBT

- Able to identify automatic thoughts
- Aware of and able to distinguish different emotions
- Accepts responsibility for change
- Understands and relates well to the rationale for CBT
- Able to develop a good collaborative relationship with the health professional
- Presents with recent or acute problems of relatively short duration
- Able to concentrate enough to focus on issues one at a time
- The patient's problems are not too severe
- Has some optimism regarding therapy

Adapted from Safran & Segal, 1990 and Safran *et al.*, 1993.

Should any patients be avoided?

Severe and major psychiatric diagnoses

A 10 Minute CBT approach in primary care is not an alternative to referral to specialist services, and may be less appropriate for patients with severe or complex mental health problems. Always assess the severity of disorders such as depression, including the presence of suicidal thoughts or plans, in order to make appropriate decisions about treatment options, and offer high quality care according to a stepped care model (NICE, 2009a).

Patients experiencing strong emotion or anger

Intense feelings during a consultation, such as severe depression or extreme anger, can distort patients' viewpoints and impair their ability to engage and collaborate with a CBT approach.

Patients who do not wish to engage with the approach

Some patients may not wish to engage with a psychological therapy such as CBT, and may prefer to try medication or an alternative talking treatment such as counselling or psychodynamic therapy. It is important to offer treatments that are appropriate and acceptable for each individual patient.

From *theory* to *practice*...

To identify whether a patient may benefit from a CBT approach, begin by subtly introducing the CBT model by asking about a patient's thoughts, feelings and behaviour in a particularly difficult situation. Try asking:

- *"What went through your mind?"*
- *"How did that make you feel?"*
- *"What did you do next?"*

Notice that some patients will understand and connect with these concepts more quickly and easily than others.

Managing time pressures

Time pressures and competing priorities can make it difficult for health professionals to consider building CBT into routine primary care consultations.

Case Example 2.1: Overcoming time pressure concerns

Dr K works in a busy surgery in an inner city location. She constantly needs to juggle the conflicting pressures of seeing patients, administrative work and home visits. She would like to learn to use CBT strategies because she thinks they might help her and her patients. However, she is very concerned about how much time it will take.

"I don't have time to use CBT. I am so busy in surgery and I already overrun quite frequently. I just couldn't cope if surgeries became any longer."

For effective time management, try to keep in mind that the aim of 10 Minute CBT is to make small incremental changes, following the patient's lead, rather than trying to achieve too much within a short time. Nevertheless, it can often be surprising to discover how much useful and interesting ground can be covered during a 10 minute consultation.

To maximise use of time, patients can be encouraged to reflect and work on their problems at home using homework tasks, which are reviewed during a later appointment. Follow-up can vary from one to several appointments and is ideally discussed and agreed in advance.

Specific consultation skills that help to manage time pressures include:
- writing a problem list
- writing down key information for the patient to review after the consultation

- choosing a specific example to focus on
- agreeing actions for the patient to try themselves in between consultations ('homework') to continue progress
- encouraging the use of self-help literature such as CBT-based books or websites.

CBT can also be used to help GPs understand and manage the consulting behaviour of some frequently attending patients. Investing time in a small number of longer consultations may help to reduce repeat attendances and save time in the longer term.

Reflecting on GP behaviour

CBT can also help health professionals to reflect on their own reactions and professional behaviour. For example, for GPs who persistently run extremely late in surgery, it can be helpful to use CBT to reflect upon why this is the case. Environmental factors such as interruptions, short appointment times and pressures to achieve multiple targets may be to blame. However, persistent lateness can sometimes also relate to internal GP factors, such as anxiety about decision-making or difficulty coping with uncertainty. Beliefs such as *'I must be 100% certain before making any decision or something terrible might happen'* can lead to anxiety and an excessive thoroughness/checking behaviour that slows down consultations considerably. *Chapter 19* on heartsink patients explores how health professionals can use CBT to understand and address some of their own personal reactions at work.

Case Example 2.1: *Continued*: alternative GP perspective on learning CBT

Dr K could try to reframe her negative thoughts and fears about learning and using CBT:

"I have limited time so I will start by trying to use the CBM in one or two consultations during surgeries that are usually less rushed"

"I am not trying to achieve miracles – using small elements of the approach can still be very helpful"

"Using 10 Minute CBT might help me to improve my management of some complex repeatedly attending patients; this could save me time in the long term!"

From *theory* to *practice*... Consider your own practice and how you might start to incorporate some brief 10 Minute CBT skills into your consultations. What will be the key obstacles to overcome? How could you use 10 Minute CBT to *improve* your time management rather than simply lengthening consultations?

Opening a 'can of worms'

Some GPs feel anxious about using CBT approaches for fear of causing harm or opening a 'can of worms' that they lack the skills to deal with appropriately. However, try to keep in mind that brief CBT in primary care does not require the GP to:

- take on extra responsibility for solving patient problems
- become a 'mini' cognitive therapist who can 'cure' complex patients in 10 minutes
- change the patient's mind or to persuade them around to the GP's own way of thinking
- use the approach with every patient in every consultation.

As described above, the key aims of 10 Minute CBT in primary care are to use the CBT model as a means of empowering patients to understand their own problems and make changes for themselves; it is largely suited to patients with mild to moderate rather than severe difficulties. This approach should be viewed as a method of guided self-help, rather than as a form of in-depth one-to-one therapy, which would require healthcare professionals to undertake more intensive training and ongoing supervision.

Whilst patients may sometimes disclose highly personal and deep-rooted emotional issues, the role of the GP in this case is not to use CBT as a therapeutic intervention, but to provide a supportive and empathic listening environment, to acknowledge and validate the patient's disclosure and to collaboratively agree the most appropriate next steps, such as referral to a specialist service.

Case Example 2.2: Dr P's story

"I was using CBT to explore why a patient felt particularly anxious with her aggressive male boss. She suddenly burst into tears and told me it was because she had been abused by her uncle when she was 11 years old. She had tried to tell her mother at the time, who had not believed the young girl's story."

"For a moment I panicked – I didn't know what to say. This lady had been to counselling and had never disclosed this to anyone. I didn't know how to react – I wanted to help her but I wasn't sure what to say."

"Then I calmed down and remembered that I didn't have to try to 'fix' her problems. I listened to her, expressed empathy for her emotional distress and reassured her that I believed her and took her story very seriously. I said that we could work together to decide what would be the appropriate next step."

"At the end of the consultation she thanked me for 'being so kind' and for listening to her. She said that she would think about what she wanted to do next and would come back *to discuss it with me again. In the end, she decided not to go to the police but attended a specialist sexual abuse counsellor. She said that being able to disclose the abuse to me had been a key first step in taking control of her past and starting to overcome her problems."*

Keeping a realistic attitude

Whilst it is not possible to carry out 'standard' CBT within 10 minute consultations, small improvements are often both possible and worthwhile. It is important to remain realistic about potential outcomes and recognise that the main aim is to increase a patient's insight and understanding of their problems, and to engage their interest in the potential for change, rather than necessarily identifying an instant solution to a patient's complex problems.

It often takes time for patients to absorb and process the new information and approach to their problems provided by CBT and so it may not be possible to end each consultation having arrived at a neat solution. In fact, ending at a more open point may encourage patients to spend time reflecting on their difficulties themselves, and can be an effective method of harnessing the time in between consultations to make progress.

Patients may leave the consultation with a small spark of new understanding, which develops further and generates change once they have had time to assimilate the information into their daily life. This can be encouraged by giving the patient a written record of the information gathered to consider in their own time.

In addition, some important outcomes from the use of the 10 Minute CBT approach may not be immediately obvious, but may arise over time – perhaps strengthening a relationship with a patient, reducing frequent attendances to surgery in a patient with health anxiety or facilitating long-term changes in a patient's life.

Learning and applying CBT skills in the general practice setting

CBT knowledge and skills can be acquired through a range of learning methods, including reading and online training modules. It is also helpful to attend practical workshops to practise and refine CBT skills in a safe environment (see www.10minuteCBT.co.uk for details). GPs with a particular interest in CBT may wish to develop more advanced skills by attending longer postgraduate training courses.

GPs can build confidence in using the approach by learning and practising the approach in stages. It is often helpful to begin by focusing on the key communication skills that are the essential building blocks to effective CBT (see *Chapters 4* and *5*).

Key learning points

Adapting CBT to primary care

- 10 Minute CBT offers a unique opportunity to offer brief CBT-based approaches in 'bite-sized' chunks to a wide variety of patients.
- Its structured approach can enhance personal and job satisfaction for health professionals, and improve patient outcomes and relationships with patients.

Using 10 Minute CBT in brief consultations

- Try not to put pressure on yourself to provide rapid or unrealistic solutions or 'cures' to a patient's problems; instead, slow down and focus on using a CBT model to understand the patient's unique difficulties in more depth.
- Work on building collaborative relationships which encourage patients to take ownership of their problems.
- Use CBT strategies which can realistically be used during a brief consultation, such as highlighting key thoughts and behaviours, using empowering explanations and encouraging behavioural change.
- Try to avoid attempting to cajole or persuade patients in the name of 'positive thinking' – this is likely to lose collaboration and undermine the therapeutic process.
- Don't be afraid to leave consultations on an 'open' note, which can encourage patients to reflect on their problems and generate changes themselves over time.

Managing time pressures

- You can use 10 Minute CBT skills on an ad hoc basis, but planning sessions in advance will allow the patient time to reflect on their problems and can help with time management; try using the approach during your first or last appointment where you feel less pressured for time.
- Remember that a surprising amount of useful and interesting ground can be covered during a 10 minute consultation.
- Key skills for effective time management include writing a problem list, writing down key information, and jointly planning 'homework' tasks for the patient to try between consultations.

Chapter 3

The cognitive-behavioural model

Introducing the cognitive-behavioural model

Using a cognitive-behavioural approach, problems can be broken down into the five areas of the CBM: thoughts, feelings, physical symptoms, behaviour and environmental factors/triggers (*Figure 3.1*). Learning to categorise people's experiences into these areas is an essential skill when learning CBT.

The CBM provides an extremely useful generic model or framework, which can easily be applied to the wide variety of problems which present in the primary care setting. For example, it could be used to understand:

- a patient with panic attacks who experiences terrifying thoughts, feelings of anxiety, and reacts with avoidance behaviour and reassurance-seeking
- a patient with a long-term physical health condition who views themself as worthless due to their illness, feels low and consequently reduces activity and avoids friends and family.

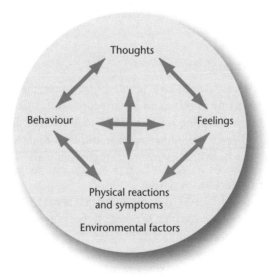

Figure 3.1: Cognitive-behavioural model (CBM)

Understanding thoughts and cognitions

What are thoughts?

'Thoughts' are the words and visual images that pass through people's minds as they make sense of the world and their experiences. They include attitudes, ideas, expectations, memories, beliefs and images.

Automatic thoughts are instantaneous, unplanned thoughts which pop up in response to events, as a running commentary. *Negative* automatic thoughts, which assume the worst in any given situation, are common in disorders such as depression and anxiety. Such negative thoughts are often exaggerated, unrealistic and unhelpful (e.g. *"I fail at absolutely everything"*), but they often *feel* highly believable to the individual, especially if linked to powerful emotions. And even if inaccurate or unfair, negative thoughts can still have serious consequences, by altering people's feelings and their subsequent behaviour.

Thoughts can take the form of both words and images. For example, a woman who develops a fear of driving may have thoughts such as *"I might crash and die if I get in the car"*. She may also experience terrifying images such as the mangled remains of a crashed car on the motorway, which markedly increase her fear of driving.

Thoughts often arise rapidly and may be difficult to catch in a particular situation. They are conscious processes, but they may occur outside the focus of immediate awareness. However, with practice, most people can learn to identify key automatic thoughts which can be associated with powerful emotions.

Chains of thoughts

Thoughts rarely occur individually – one thought about a particular issue commonly leads to others in rapid succession. Imagine that Sally, a 25 year old student, is waiting for her friend to arrive for dinner. She feels sad and depressed because she has begun to think that her friend does not really like her. She may have a sequence of thoughts such as:

⇒ my friend is late for dinner
⇒ she probably had something more interesting or important to do
⇒ this must mean that she thinks I am boring
⇒ she probably doesn't really like me
⇒ no one ever likes me
⇒ there is no point in inviting anyone to visit me – they won't want to come
⇒ it must be because I am a really horrible, boring person
⇒ my life is meaningless and empty.

Such a cascade is often very rapid – within a few seconds – and Sally may not be consciously aware of all of the steps. However, rather than simply feeling a little disappointed or put out that her friend has not yet arrived, she begins to feel depressed and low because the cascade of thoughts has led to the conclusion that she is boring and that her life is meaningless.

CBT teaches patients to view their thoughts as merely *hypotheses* or *guesses* to be tested against reality, rather than absolute fact. It may not be possible to alter an immediate, automatic thought which arises in response to a challenging situation. However, patients *can* learn to identify and test out whether their automatic thoughts represent a realistic assessment or whether another perspective may be more accurate and helpful. This process of identifying a more balanced perspective may also reduce negative feelings.

From *theory* to *practice*: Identifying thoughts	When people become distressed, take time to try to fully understand the cascade of thoughts that underlie the emotional reaction. Listen carefully and gently ask questions such as: *"What was going through your mind just then?"* *"What is it about this situation that really upsets you?"* *"I noticed that you became really [sad] just then, what were you thinking?"*

Feelings and emotions

In CBT terminology, 'feelings' are viewed as emotions or moods, such as happy, excited, angry, sad, frustrated, embarrassed or fearful. Some common negative feelings include:

- **sadness and loss**, e.g. feeling low, down, unhappy, depressed, miserable, sad, fed up, disappointed
- **guilt and shame**, e.g. ashamed, guilty, embarrassed, humiliated, mortified
- **anxiety and fear**, e.g. nervous, tense, frightened, anxious, worried, afraid, scared, panicky, terrified, petrified
- **anger and hurt**, e.g. annoyed, irritated, frustrated, cross, exasperated, angry, furious, mad, livid, infuriated, hurt

People use many different words to describe their feelings. For example, feeling 'upset' could represent feelings of sadness, hurt, anger or guilt. It is important to clarify the meaning by asking:

"What did feeling 'upset' mean for you in this situation? Are there any other ways to describe how you felt?"

Some people have difficulty in accurately identifying or expressing their feelings. They may view the expression of emotions as a sign of 'weakness' or may be attempting to suppress very powerful negative emotions for fear of being overwhelmed. In these cases, people can be slowly encouraged to accept, identify and monitor different feelings. Alternatively, it may be more helpful to focus more on thoughts and behaviour than on labelling emotions.

Rating feelings

Patients can learn to rate the intensity of their feelings, for example, on a scale from 0–100. It can be helpful to use a visual rating scale for this (*Figure 3.2*):

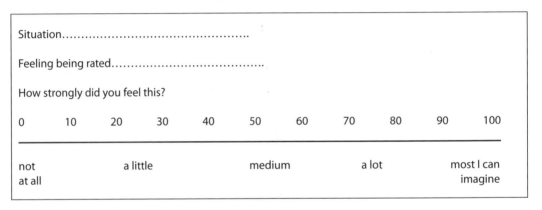

Figure 3.2: Rating scale for intensity of feelings (adapted from Greenberger & Padesky, 1995a)

Monitoring the intensity of feelings usually shows that they fluctuate widely over a period of time. This can be helpful in depression, where patients often overlook or discount positive experiences and hold beliefs such as: "*I always feel terrible; I'm constantly depressed*".

Identifying even minor fluctuations in mood begins to challenge the depressed person's thought that life is *completely terrible*. This opens up the possibility that there may be some small positive things in life *already* and that the patient's task is to build upon these. This can offer hope and encouragement and make the task of overcoming depression seem less overwhelming.

It is also useful to record any changes in intensity of feelings when the patient tries a new strategy to cope with their problems. For example, a depressed person could record how they feel before and after going for a walk. This helps reinforce the benefit of particular behaviours and offers an objective measure of the patient's progress. Even a small reduction in negative feelings, perhaps from 80 down to 60, still represents an important improvement in mood.

The relationship between thoughts and feelings

Separating thoughts from feelings

Learning to differentiate thoughts and feelings is a core CBT skill which is essential for both health professionals and patients to acquire. As a general rule, feelings and emotions can usually be described in one word (e.g. anger, sadness, fear). If it takes more than one word to describe a mood, this is likely to be describing a thought rather than a feeling.

In the English language, it is common to insert the word 'feel' into a statement which is actually a thought. It is usually used to indicate that the speaker is aware that the thought or belief is their own opinion or perspective. For example, a patient may say:

"I feel that my husband is really upset with me"

This statement is a *thought* not a feeling. Health professionals can help patients to learn to differentiate between the two by reflecting back the patient's words and asking for any associated emotions. Be prepared to ask several times if the patient does not understand your meaning, for example, by saying:

"How does it make you feel when you think that your husband is upset with you?"

The patient may reply:

"I feel that he is starting to drift away and that he might want to leave me"

Again, this is another thought. You could react to this by asking again:

"And how do you feel about the idea that your husband may be drifting away from you and might want to leave you?"

The patient may then respond by describing her feelings about the situation:

"I feel anxious and terrified. I don't know how I would cope on my own"

Remember, it is usually unhelpful to challenge or question the validity of a patient's feelings. These are subjective experiences that can only be felt and described by that individual. However, it may be possible to change any associated unhelpful thoughts or behaviours, which may indirectly alter the negative feelings.

Connections between thoughts and feelings

There is usually a logical relationship between people's thoughts and feelings.

For example, in depression, the characteristic thoughts are negatively biased views of themselves, of the world and the future.

"I'm useless, nothing ever goes right for me and it will never get any better..."

In anxiety, thoughts tend to be biased towards overestimating the threat of danger, as well as underestimating their own ability to cope with the problem.

"Something terrible might happen and it will be a complete disaster..."

In anger, thoughts tend to be about a perceived unfairness or breaking of some implicit or explicit rule, and can involve a hostile intent.

"They should not have done that, it's not right..."

There is a reciprocal relationship between thoughts and feelings. In other words, thinking negatively is likely to make people feel bad and feeling low will also make people think more negatively. The more intensely we experience a particular emotion, the more extreme the associated thinking is likely to be.

Identifying a patient's thoughts and feelings about a particular event can help health professionals develop *empathy* for their individual reactions to life experiences (*Box 3.1*). It becomes possible to put ourselves into the patient's shoes by imagining: *"If I believed that then I would also expect to feel..."*

Box 3.1

Linking thoughts and feelings

In the following exercise, cover the right hand column and consider which feelings you might expect to coincide with the following list of thoughts:

Thought	Possible feeling(s)
"What if I give a terrible speech to my colleagues? It might go down like a lead balloon and they will think I'm incompetent."	Anxiety/fear
"I'm worthless. No one wants me."	Sadness/depression
"My son failed to get to university. It's my fault. I'm a bad parent."	Guilt
"I showed myself up in public by swearing at those people."	Shame
"He shouldn't interrupt me. He's a thoughtless idiot."	Anger

From *theory* to *practice*...

Make sure you clearly understand the difference between thoughts and feelings. Next time a patient expresses a particular emotion, try to develop a curiosity about what thoughts might underpin their feelings. Gently explore with genuine interest to try to understand why they feel that way.

Can you identify the key thoughts that are responsible for the difficult feelings? Does this make logical sense? If not then you may need to explore a little further.

Don't worry at this stage about what to 'do' with the thoughts once you have identified them. Simply reflect them back to the patient and express empathy for the patient's distress.

Case Example 3.1: Separating thoughts and feelings in action

Jane is a 30 year old single parent. In the following dialogue, she discusses some of her concerns about her 10 year old son Adam. Jane is struggling to juggle working full-time with bringing up her son. She is feeling increasingly depressed and low.

GP "What has been going on with Adam that has been getting you down?"

Jane "Well, he has been misbehaving at school lately. I got called in to see his teacher last week. He was doing so well last year, and now he is near the bottom of the class."

GP "I see. That must be quite a worry for you."

Jane "Oh yes, it is. And with work being so busy right now, I'm at the end of my tether. I feel so low and tired. Everything is a complete mess. When I went to see his teacher, I'm sure she blamed me for everything."

GP "What makes you say that?"

Jane "Well, I was 15 minutes late to see her because I got held up at work. She must have thought that I'm a terrible mother. And then she asked if there were any problems at home. Later on I started thinking about it. Maybe she's right, I am a bad mother. I've been too busy at work to give him the time he needs. I've failed and now his school work is suffering. I feel so useless." (Looks very tearful)

Jane's problems can be broken down into:

Situation / events   Adam misbehaving at school and at home

Adam's performance at school going downhill

Work being busy

Being called in to see Adam's teacher

Thoughts	"I'm at the end of my tether"
	"Everything is a complete mess"
	"Adam's teacher thinks I'm a terrible mother"
	"I am a bad mother"
	"I've failed"
	"I'm useless"
Feelings	Low
Physical reactions	Tired
	Tearful

Breaking the problem down in this way enables Jane to separate the problems with Adam and his school work from her own thoughts of inadequacy and feelings of low mood. Problem-solving techniques may help to resolve some of the complex difficulties she is facing in her life, such as coping as a single mother with a busy job. It may also be helpful for her to look at some of her negative thinking and behaviours which may be worsening her confidence and lowering her mood.

CBT and positive thinking

CBT is *not* simply thinking positively. Overly positive thinking can be just as unhelpful as excessively negative thinking. For example, if a patient keeps telling herself to *"Look on the bright side – everything will be fine"*, there is a risk that her problems may actually get worse because she is not doing anything useful to solve them.

CBT encourages *realistic* thinking. This means taking into account both positive and negative aspects of any problem. By taking this broad perspective, people are better equipped to deal with the issues that they face in life.

The role of behaviour

'Behaviour' refers to observable actions that people carry out – what they *do*. Certain behaviours are characteristic of particular emotional disorders, and generally act to maintain or worsen problems as a vicious cycle. Common unhelpful behaviours include:

- **depression**: reduced activity, excessive rest, withdrawal from social activity
- **anxiety**: avoidance or 'escape' from anxiety-provoking situations, reassurance-seeking, safety behaviours designed to minimise or protect the self from a particular threat.

These behaviours will be discussed in more detail in the clinical chapters of *Section C*.

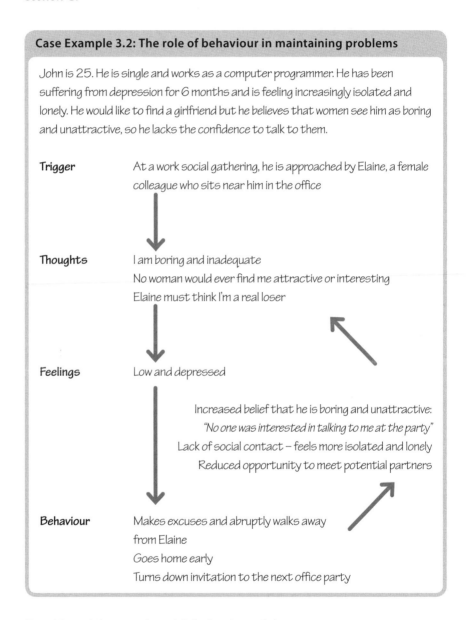

Case Example 3.2: The role of behaviour in maintaining problems

John is 25. He is single and works as a computer programmer. He has been suffering from depression for 6 months and is feeling increasingly isolated and lonely. He would like to find a girlfriend but he believes that women see him as boring and unattractive, so he lacks the confidence to talk to them.

Trigger   At a work social gathering, he is approached by Elaine, a female colleague who sits near him in the office

Thoughts   I am boring and inadequate
                   No woman would ever find me attractive or interesting
                   Elaine must think I'm a real loser

Feelings   Low and depressed

                   Increased belief that he is boring and unattractive:
                   "No one was interested in talking to me at the party"
                   Lack of social contact – feels more isolated and lonely
                   Reduced opportunity to meet potential partners

Behaviour   Makes excuses and abruptly walks away
                   from Elaine
                   Goes home early
                   Turns down invitation to the next office party

Breaking vicious cycles with behavioural changes

Changing behaviour can be one of the most powerful ways to break negative cycles and improve a patient's symptoms. It is possible to *behave* differently, irrespective of how we think or feel. This is a very powerful strategy for making positive change. Altering behaviour can have a marked impact on all other areas of the CBM, including thoughts, feelings and even physical symptoms.

Promoting behaviour change is a particularly useful and effective strategy to use within the time limitations of the primary care setting. The patient can be encouraged to behave *'as if'* they feel better or differently rather than waiting to feel less depressed or anxious before making changes in behaviour. We will look in more detail at how to encourage behavioural change in *Chapter 8*.

From *theory* to *practice*... Focus closely on the impact of behaviour on people's experiences. What kinds of helpful or unhelpful behaviour do you notice? Does any behaviour result in a 'vicious cycle' which makes problems worse? What happens if they change this behaviour, even in very small ways?

Physical reactions and symptoms

Emotional reactions are associated with a range of physical and biological reactions. Reading a scary book can lead to a rapid heart rate or sweaty palms as the reader imagines a frightening scene. Thinking about an exciting or enjoyable future event can lead to tingles down the spine or butterflies in the stomach.

Physical symptoms also play a key role in sustaining problems such as panic disorder and depression. In panic disorder, patients tend to misinterpret harmless anxiety-related physical symptoms such as a racing heart or rapid breathing, as indicating a potentially severe or life-threatening problem such as having a heart attack. This terrifying thought simply increases anxiety as a vicious cycle (*Figure 3.3*).

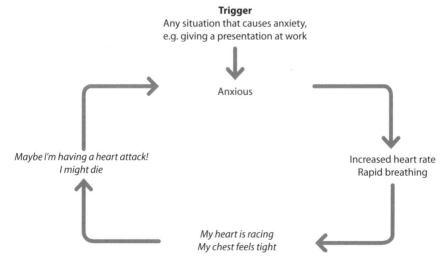

Trigger
Any situation that causes anxiety,
e.g. giving a presentation at work

Anxious

Increased heart rate
Rapid breathing

Maybe I'm having a heart attack!
I might die

My heart is racing
My chest feels tight

Figure 3.3: Vicious cycles in anxiety

Physical aspects of emotional disorders are important, because many patients will initially present to primary care with physical rather than psychological symptoms, such as tiredness, headaches, bowel symptoms, or pain. In addition, patients suffering from chronic physical disease, with the associated problems of pain, functional impairment and disability, are at increased risk of developing depression and anxiety. Depression exacerbates the pain and distress associated with physical illnesses and adversely affects outcomes, including reducing life expectancy and increasing any functional impairment. Depression is also a risk factor in the development of physical illness, including cardiovascular disease (NICE, 2009b).

From *theory* to *practice*…	Start to notice the connections between physical symptoms, thoughts and feelings. In one or two patients with emotional distress, remember to ask about associated physical changes.
	In one or two patients presenting with physical symptoms, try to identify what they think and feel about their symptoms or their disorder.

Environment, social circumstances and culture

Environmental factors influence our emotional health and ability to cope with adverse life circumstances and events. These factors include early childhood experiences and social and cultural factors, and can make individuals more vulnerable to developing emotional disorders in certain circumstances.

Nevertheless, it is also important to keep in mind that emotional disorders are not *inevitable* consequences of financial hardship or other social problems. Patients may still benefit greatly from CBT approaches to their problems and these can be an effective approach for people from all walks of life.

Early experiences

Early childhood experiences shape people's beliefs about themselves, others and the rest of the world. This can contribute to the formation of deep-rooted beliefs known as 'rules' and 'core beliefs'. The presence of particular underlying beliefs can help to explain why particular individuals develop depression or anxiety in the face of specific stressful life circumstances; more about these types of belief will be covered in *Chapter 10*.

Case Example 3.3: The role of early childhood experiences in shaping core beliefs

Roger grew up with a critical and distant father. If Roger did badly at school, his father would react angrily saying: "If you fail at school, you will never get anywhere in life". Roger worked harder, hoping to gain his father's approval. He achieved high grades in most subjects but his father would always notice when he was not top of the class. "You only came second in maths. You have to try harder..." No matter how hard he worked, his father continued to comment on his faults. Consequently, Roger developed deep-seated 'core beliefs' that he was inadequate, a failure and that he was stupid.

Later in life, despite becoming a successful banker, Roger still retained some of these beliefs about himself. He became a perfectionist, believing that "As long as I am successful in every way then I am OK. But, coming second in anything means total failure." These 'rules' drove him to overwork and become highly competitive in everything he did. As long as he remained successful, he felt confident in himself.

However, along with several of his colleagues, Roger was unexpectedly made redundant from work. This life event triggered the reactivation of his negative beliefs about his own failure and stupidity. Given these underlying beliefs, it is unsurprising that Roger found it difficult to cope with the perceived 'failure' of redundancy. In this situation, his reactivated core beliefs resulted in a cascade of negative thoughts and feelings, which gradually developed into depression.

Social and environmental circumstances

The social and environmental circumstances of daily life also play a major role in determining individual people's vulnerability to emotional disorders and distress. People are much more likely to feel unhappy and low in situations where they feel:

- unloved or uncared for
- an outsider – not part of any group
- unsupported or abandoned
- rejected by others
- unattractive to self or others
- unappreciated or not valued by others
- having low status or experiencing a loss of status
- lacking a supporting network: friends and family
- lacking social support, e.g. religious or local community.

Life events

Experiencing a major life event makes individuals more likely to develop an emotional disorder. Important life events include the death of a close relative or friend, moving house, loss of a job, the breakdown of a relationship, or the birth of a child.

Individual vulnerability to developing an emotional disorder in response to particular life events will be influenced by several factors, including previous life experiences and core beliefs, and an individual's personal 'resilience'. This is an ability to cope with or bounce back from difficult situations. Developing resilience can enhance people's ability to cope with adverse life circumstances.

Cultural and other social factors

People are also influenced by many other factors including cultural/ethnic backgrounds, religion, family beliefs, gender roles, work environments and the media.

Cultural factors play a powerful role in shaping people's norms and values, and their beliefs about themselves and the world. Health professionals must be sensitive to the possibility of different cultural perspectives and norms. It is possible to incorrectly label a patient's beliefs as 'unhelpful' when these beliefs actually represent a normal cultural perspective for that individual.

From *theory* to *practice*...	If you regularly see patients from a particular cultural group, it can be helpful to educate yourself about that culture in order to better understand the context of patient experiences. However, you must also try to avoid making assumptions about the beliefs held by people from particular cultures. Instead, help the individual to evaluate their beliefs within the context of their own personal and cultural perspective.

Developing a 'case formulation'

The CBM can act as the starting point for developing an individual *case formulation*. This involves creating an individualised map or overview of an individual's problems in terms of cognitive behavioural theory and is a key element of the therapeutic process in CBT.

Developing a case formulation provides a framework to make sense of complex problems. The process is often therapeutic and beneficial in its own right, because it promotes the patient's understanding and insight into their problems. It is usually collaboratively shared with the patient to facilitate this. A case formulation helps to guide the therapy process and enables ongoing CBT strategies to be tailored to the patient's individual needs and problems.

Westbrook *et al.* (2007) define a case formulation as using the CBT model to develop:
- a description of the current problem(s)
- an account of why and how these problems may have developed
- an analysis of the key processes that maintain the problem(s).

A general model of case formulation is illustrated in *Figure 3.4*.

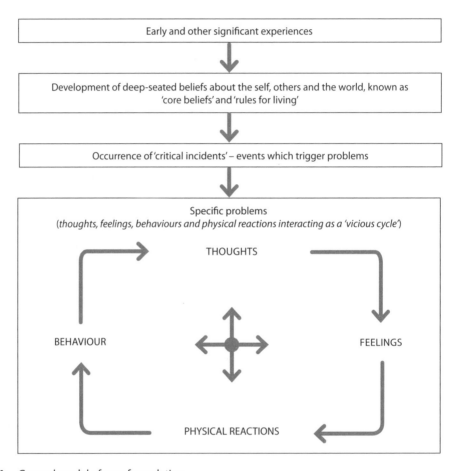

Figure 3.4: General model of case formulation

<table>
<tr><td>**From *theory* to *practice*...**</td><td>Try breaking down one of your own personal difficulties into different areas of the CBM:

Thoughts, feelings, behaviour, physical reactions and environmental factors.

What is the impact of looking at the problem in this way? Are you able to learn anything new from this different perspective?</td></tr>
</table>

Key learning points

- The CBM provides a simple framework to make sense of an individual patient's problems.
- Try to discuss all five areas of the CBM when assessing any mental or physical health problem. This does not have to be part of a formal CBT approach, but can simply involve asking about thoughts, feelings, behaviour and symptoms in a particular situation.
- Make brief notes if necessary to help your memory. You can also give this information to the patient at the end to help them reflect after the consultation.
- **Thoughts** – explore the thoughts which underlie a negative emotional reaction. Be curious and use Socratic questioning to gently explore the meaning that the patient attributes to difficult experiences. Use this information to build empathy and improve your relationship.
- **Feelings** – feelings represent emotional reactions such as sad, anxious, angry, etc. Ensure that you are confident distinguishing between feelings (which can usually be described in one word) and thoughts (which represent an evaluation of a situation). Consider using a simple emotional rating scale to monitor fluctuations in the intensity of feelings.
- **Behaviour** – ask the patient what they are doing (or not doing) in response to their problems. This is one of the most important areas to discuss in depth because simple behaviour changes are often the most effective starting point for breaking vicious cycles and making positive change. Encourage patients to behave 'as if' they feel differently, rather than waiting to feel better before making any changes.
- **Physical symptoms** – remember to ask about physical aspects of emotional disorders, such as tiredness in depression, which may contribute to a patient's problems by increasing inactivity, as well as distressing physical symptoms associated with physical illnesses and long-term conditions.
- **Social and environmental factors** – ask about any relevant social and environmental factors, including early life experiences, cultural and social factors and major life events. CBT can enhance people's resilience and ability to cope with adverse environmental circumstances.

Chapter 4

Introducing a cognitive-behavioural approach to patients

Getting started

It is important to give patients a clear rationale for using a CBT approach, because it may be different to anything they have encountered in the past. This also develops a partnership with your patient who must understand the model in order to take an active role in their own treatment.

Begin by emphasising that your principal aim is to understand and make sense of problems rather than to offer an instant 'cure'. A CBT approach should be a 'no-lose' strategy, which avoids any sense of blame – for either GP or patient – if it proves to be unhelpful.

> "I would like to understand more about your problems and how they are affecting your life."

> "Some people find it helpful to look at their problems from a different perspective. This involves talking through all of the different aspects of your problems. You might also discover some new ways to cope better with your particular difficulties."

Using a written CBM chart

The 10 Minute CBT approach is most effective if the information gathered is written down, with one copy kept for the GP's records and another given to the patient. You could use a CBM chart to gather this information (see *Figure 4.1*). Written information can be copied and scanned into computer records, or held in a folder in a secure location. Generally, only a brief summary needs to be entered directly into a patient's notes, along with any particular outcomes or treatment issued.

Writing down information can improve communication with patients, provided it is used in a sensitive, open and collaborative way, and eye contact is maintained in between making notes (*Box 4.1*). Sit with the piece of paper positioned between clinician and patient, with both able to see it clearly.

Recent example:	
Thoughts	**Feelings**
Behaviour	**Physical symptoms / biology**
Environmental factors / triggers	
Agreed actions / homework	

Figure 4.1: CBM chart to use in consultations

Box 4.1

Benefits of writing down relevant information

- It helps patients remember key points from the consultation. This is particularly important for patients experiencing depression or anxiety, who often have difficulties with concentration and memory
- Seeing their own words in black and white helps patients to gain a broader perspective and to think more flexibly about their problems
- A written overview highlights any links between different areas of a patient's problems; these can be drawn as arrows on the CBM chart
- Writing slows the process of information gathering and gives the consultation more structure and focus
- Written notes enable the GP to reflect back accurate summaries of the information, using the patient's own words

Use of written records: what to say

> "It is important for me to remember what you say, so I would like to write down the main points. We can discuss whatever I write and you can take away a copy after the consultation. How do you feel about this...?"

You can also use written records to summarise and clarify important points:

> "You said that you felt 'hurt' and 'angry' – I am going to write that down. Is that OK?"

> "You have given me lots of information here which seems important to note down. Let's go over the key points..."

From *theory* to *practice*…	Try writing information from patients down, using the CBM as a structured framework. Treat it as a 'behavioural experiment'.
	What happens? Try to determine in which situations and with which patients using written notes is most useful. Remember to ask the patient whether they found it helpful as well.

Talking through the CBM

It is usually helpful to begin by talking about the area that the patient is already focused on as their presenting complaint. For example, if a patient is complaining of anxiety then you might say:

> "You mentioned that you get very anxious and panicky, so I will make a note of that on this chart. I would like to talk about some of the ways that you think and react when you feel so anxious. Can you give me a recent example of when you felt like this...?"

This shows the patient that you are interested in what they see as the major problem and helps to build trust. It will also facilitate the later exploration of other aspects of the problem, such as behavioural or cognitive factors, which the patient may not initially view as being relevant. This is particularly important in problems like health anxiety, where the patient is very fixed on one particular aspect of their problem – their physical symptoms. In this case, begin by reviewing the physical symptoms which are causing concern.

Discussing thoughts

Accurately understanding people's thoughts is central to understanding their reactions to particular situations and events. Be specific in recording thoughts and worries, by asking for recent examples of problems, e.g. a recent panic attack or a time when the patient felt really low.

Make sure that you write down the patient's *own words* rather than summarising or paraphrasing, which may not resonate with their actual experiences and risks losing the emotional connection with the patient. Remember also to use the first person, for example, by writing *"I am a failure"* rather than *"Thinking about being a failure".*

Some helpful questions to identify a patient's thoughts are given in *Box 4.2.*

Box 4.2

Questions to help identify negative automatic thoughts

- *"What was going through your mind...? What were you thinking?"*
- *"What is the worst bit about this situation? What is so bad about it?"*
- *"What does this say about yourself, your life or your future?"*
- *"How do you see yourself, your behaviour or your performance?"*
- *"Were you afraid that something might happen? What would be the worst thing?"*
- *"How do you think others thought or felt about you in that situation? What does that mean to you?"*
- *"Did you have any particular memories or images?"*

Use a Socratic questioning style

Health professionals should demonstrate an attitude of curiosity and genuine interest in the patient's perspective, and use an appropriate questioning style, which does not feel like an aggressive interrogation. This will often generate a similar enthusiasm in the patient, which encourages them to reflect upon important problems. Useful questions may involve asking the patient to reflect and clarify their meaning, such as:

"I wonder what makes that feel so difficult for you...?"

"Can you help me understand why that made you feel so sad..?"

Thoughts should reflect the patient's key emotions (and vice versa) and this relationship should make logical sense to the listener. If you don't quite feel you fully understand, continue to gently ask questions:

"I would like to understand but I'm not quite with you. Can you explain what that means for you?"

Case Example 4.1: Identifying thoughts

Alison is a 25 year old hairdresser who has been suffering from stress and anxiety for six months. She used to be part of a large group of friends, but has recently become anxious about being in groups. She has begun to make excuses to avoid meeting them and has become more isolated in her daily life.

GP	"You said that you felt very anxious just before you were due to go and meet your friends. What was going through your mind at that moment?"
Alison	"I didn't want to go because the whole evening would probably be a disaster."
GP	"What might happen to make the whole evening a disaster?"
Alison	"Well, I might say something really stupid in front of the group, or I might not say anything at all."
GP	"Supposing that did happen – that you said something stupid in front of the group, or you didn't have anything to say – what would be so bad about that?"
Alison	"I suppose I worry that my friends would laugh at me. They might think less of me. And if I don't say anything at all, they would think I am boring."
GP	"OK, I would like to summarise what I heard you say. Last Thursday evening you were due to meet some friends. Before going out, you were feeling very anxious and you were thinking: 'The whole evening might be a disaster. I might say something stupid in front of the group or not say anything at all. My friends might laugh at me and think less of me. If I don't say anything they will think I am boring.' Is that right? Is there anything you would like to change?"
Alison	"That's right. I hadn't really thought of it like that before. It made me feel really tense and uptight before I went out."

Notice how the GP simply listened and recorded Alison's thoughts, word for word, *without* trying to question or challenge them. Once both Alison and GP fully understand all five areas of the CBM in relation to this problem, only then is it helpful to consider challenging or reframing thoughts.

From *theory* to *practice*…

Make a note of some key questions to ask patients about their thoughts. You may sometimes be surprised at the answers you receive!

These questions are a good way to understand more about a patient's experiences, attitudes and beliefs even without discussing all five areas of the CBM.

Discussing feelings

It is important to identify the feelings that cause patients major emotional distress. Try to stay focused and relate feelings to specific thoughts and situations:

"When you start to think ... how does that make you feel?"

"How did you feel in that situation...?"

If you simply wish to gain a broad understanding of the patient's feelings and other experiences, it is sometimes helpful to take a more general approach:

"Can you tell me a bit about how you are generally and how you are feeling?"

Patients are not always easily able to articulate their feelings and so if a patient has difficulty in identifying their feelings, one option is to suggest the likely *opposite* reaction:

"Did you feel very happy and relaxed in that situation?"

The patient will often respond quickly to correct the 'error':

"Oh no, I felt really stressed and uptight."

This opens up the discussion and gives the GP an opportunity to discuss any associated thoughts and behaviours.

"What was going through your mind that was making you feel stressed and uptight?"

As a last resort, if a patient is really struggling to identify their feelings, the clinician can make one or two suggestions. However, you must also accept that these are *guesses* and may be inaccurate.

"Some people find that this kind of situation makes them feel fed up or down, could that be true for you? If not, what might be more accurate?"

"I could imagine that thinking 'I am such a failure' might make someone feel very low. Is that true for you?"

You can also reflect back to patients any particular feelings that you have observed. Again, it is important to be flexible and be aware that you may have incorrectly labelled a particular feeling.

"This pain really seems to make you angry."

"You seem very sad and low when you say that."

It is always important to express empathy for a patient's unpleasant feelings and experiences:

"It must be really difficult to feel so anxious."

Looking at behaviour

It is important to spend time identifying a patient's helpful and unhelpful behaviours and coping strategies and how these relate to other areas of the CBM. Begin by simply asking the patient how they behave in particular situations.

> *"What happens when you feel anxious? What do you do then?"*

For patients with anxiety, it is also helpful to identify any safety behaviours that they are carrying out to try to avoid feelings of anxiety and worry.

> *"Do you do anything to stop yourself from getting anxious?"*

It is also important to find out if there is anything that the patient is *not doing* or avoiding. Try asking the patient to compare their current behaviour to that of other times in their lives or to other people's reactions:

> *"What are you doing differently now that you feel so low? How was life before this?"*

> *"How might you behave differently if you felt happier and more relaxed?"*

> *"Do you know anyone who would react differently? What would they do?"*

It is sometimes useful to discuss the specific thoughts and fears that underlie certain behaviours. This helps to make sense of reactions which may initially seem self-defeating and difficult to understand.

> *"What is the worst thing that could happen if you hadn't taken that action to cope with your symptoms?"*

From *theory* to *practice*...	Remember to include questions about behaviour when discussing problems with patients.
	Try to discover *unhelpful* behaviours, which may worsen problems, as well as *helpful* coping strategies, which can be encouraged. What underlying thoughts, fears or beliefs are driving these behaviours?
	Can you identify any unhelpful behaviour in one or two patients with physical disorders such as back pain or diabetes, or a patient with mild to moderate anxiety or depression?

Physical symptoms

Physical reactions also play an important role in the CBM.

> *"I would like to briefly review how this is affecting you physically. Can you remind me which physical symptoms you commonly experience?"*

It is often useful to identify the patient's physical reactions during a particular situation.

"How did you feel physically when you were feeling anxious? What did you notice in your body?

Discussing physical symptoms is particularly important where unhelpful beliefs exist about the *meaning* of symptoms, such as in panic attacks or health anxiety.

"It will be helpful for me to get an overview of all of your different symptoms."

Remember to express empathy for any unpleasant or distressing physical experiences, without jumping prematurely to try to explain or discount the patient's experiences.

"It must be really distressing to be in so much pain."

You can also spend some time discussing the patient's underlying fears and beliefs about the meaning of their symptoms.

"What is the most distressing part about experiencing the pain?"

"What do you think that having this headache means? Do you have any thoughts about what might be causing it?"

"What went through your mind when you noticed the tightness in your chest?"

Negative thoughts or beliefs about how to respond to particular symptoms may also result in unhelpful behaviours, such as excessive resting with back pain.

"How do you react when you experience the pain? What might happen if you did not?"

It is also important to understand the impact of particular symptoms on the patient's life. You should also ask if they fear any possible future changes.

"How do these symptoms affect your life? How does that make you feel emotionally?"

"Do you see yourself differently now that you have gone through the mastectomy?"

"Are you concerned that something may change or worsen in the future?"

Try to finish with a summary of the physical symptoms and any related thoughts and feelings. This highlights the links between physical and psychological aspects of problems *without* suggesting that physical symptoms are 'all in the patient's mind' and somehow not 'real'.

"You mentioned that you are experiencing some very unpleasant symptoms, which are making your life really difficult. You are suffering from headaches, dizziness and occasional tingling in the feet. The dizziness is the most unpleasant symptom. You had a bout of dizziness yesterday, and when it happened, you began to think: 'Maybe I have got a brain tumour' which made you feel very anxious."

More detail about discussing physical symptoms in patients with health anxiety and medically unexplained symptoms is covered in *Chapter 14*.

From *theory* to *practice*…	Choose one or two patients with distressing physical symptoms. Review their symptoms and identify any underlying fears and beliefs about the meaning of symptoms.
	How does experiencing the symptoms affect the patient's life? Do they fear that this could change or worsen in the future?
	What kinds of feelings are associated with these thoughts? Does this affect how the patient behaves?

Social and environmental factors

It is important to identify any social and environmental stressors which may contribute to a patient's difficulties (*Box 4.3*).

Box 4.3	**Social and environmental factors**
	• Are there problems with any important relationships (family, friends, neighbours)?
	• *"Do you have enough support?"*
	• *"Do you have someone to talk to about problems?"*
	• Are there demands at home, such as looking after children or other relatives?
	• Are there money troubles?
	• Are there any particular problems with housing or the home environment?
	• *"Are you unemployed or unable to work?"*
	• Are there difficulties at work?

It is useful to give patients a rationale for asking about their personal life circumstances:

"It may help to understand anything going on in your life which may be making you feel upset and making your symptoms worse."

It may also be important to identify and understand whether particular situations act as triggers for problems:

"Do the panic attacks arise in any specific situations?"

"What is it about this situation that you find so difficult? What is the worst thing that could happen?"

Summarising what you have heard

Always try to end your discussion with a brief summary which highlights the key points of the discussion. Use your written notes as a prompt and ensure that you use the patient's own words.

Finding relationships between different areas of a problem can help identify new coping strategies or solutions. So, try to highlight any vicious cycles or links between the key physical symptoms, thoughts, feelings and behaviours that you have identified. You could also ask a 'handover' question which asks the patient to reflect on the information and come up with their own conclusions. The use of summarising and handover questions will be discussed in more detail in *Chapter 5*.

Key learning points

- Always give patients a clear rationale for the CBT approach.
- Use a written CBM chart to record thoughts, feelings and behaviours; give a copy to the patient to help them remember the discussion.
- Finish with a summary and ask the patient what they have learned from the discussion.

	Remember	Ask
Thoughts	Show a genuine curiosity and interest in hearing the patient's story, and keep a gentle tone that avoids the consultation seeming like an 'interrogation'. Use the patient's own words when recording and discussing their thoughts.	*"What was going through your mind…? What were you thinking?"* *"What is the worst bit about this situation?"* *"What does this mean about you?"* *"What is the worst thing that might happen?"*

	Remember	Ask
Feelings	Ask about the feelings associated with specific situations and thoughts. Always express empathy for a patient's emotional distress.	*"How did that make you feel?"* *"What emotions came up at that point?"* *"That must be very difficult..."*
Physical symptoms	Ask about any physical symptoms associated with emotional problems. For physical health conditions, jointly write a detailed list of symptoms. Ask about health beliefs and fears about the meaning of particular distressing symptoms.	*"What symptoms arise when you get anxious?"* *"What do you worry that they might mean?"* *"I'd like to make a list of the main symptoms that are bothering you..."*
Behaviour	Identifying unhelpful behaviour patterns is a key aspect of finding and breaking vicious cycles and making positive change. Try to find out what thoughts or fears are driving unhelpful behaviours.	*"What did you do? What did you do next?"* *"What are you no longer doing because of this problem?"* *"Are you doing anything to protect yourself from harm or check for problems?"*
Social and environmental factors	Ask about key environmental and social factors that are having a negative impact on patient's health and wellbeing. Also ask about environmental triggers for problems such as panic attacks.	*"Are there any particular difficulties in your life that might be part of the problem?"* *"Has anything happened in the past to make you particularly worried about this?"*

Chapter 5

Communication skills for CBT

Effective communication in CBT

Effective communication, which builds a strong 'therapeutic alliance', is essential, although not sufficient, for the CBT process. The building blocks of effective communication include:

- warmth, concern and genuineness
- mutual trust and respect
- developing rapport
- showing compassion
- adhering to ethical standards, such as privacy, confidentiality and honesty
- giving information about your role and its limitations
- ability to adapt personal style so that it 'meshes' with that of the patient
- avoiding unhelpful interpersonal behaviours (e.g. impatience or insincerity).

Health professionals should convey their genuine interest in exploring a patient's problems, using encouraging body language, maintaining eye contact, nodding, and the use of silence when appropriate. The tone of voice and style of questioning are important to gain a patient's trust. For example, *"Why...?"* questions can seem intrusive and more threatening than opening phrases such as *"How...?"* or *"Tell me about..."*.

Using open questions will encourage the patient to contribute to the discussion. These include broad open questions to establish the patient's main areas of concern, and more focused specific open questions to clarify important information about key problem areas:

> *"How does that affect you...?"*

> *"Can you give me an example...?"*

> *"What was it about that situation that really bothered you...?"*

The therapeutic relationship in CBT

The quality of the relationship between CBT therapist and patient is important, with evidence suggesting it is strongly linked to the therapeutic outcome

(Horvath & Symonds, 1991; Orlinsky *et al.*, 1994). A therapeutic alliance is usually considered to have three aspects (Roth & Pilling, 2007):

- the relationship or bond between professional and patient
- agreement on the goals of therapy
- agreement on the change process and the techniques/methods to be used.

Specific elements of the relationship may be especially important in predicting a good outcome from therapy. In particular, the degree to which the patient is involved and engaged in the session is crucial. A patient is more likely to do well if they are engaged with the therapeutic task, offer suggestions about treatment, interact warmly and trust the therapist (Westbrook *et al.*, 2007). Completion of homework tasks is also a key predictor of benefit from CBT (Burns & Nolen-Hoeksema, 1991).

Interpersonal difficulties between health professional and patient, which can be viewed as 'ruptures' in the therapeutic relationship, are covered in more detail in *Chapter 19* on heartsink patients.

Building collaborative relationships

Collaboration involves building a partnership where GP and patient work together as a team to understand problems, set goals and work on solutions. Collaborative relationships are promoted through the use of consultation skills such as negotiating an agenda, jointly planning session content, actively obtaining patient feedback, giving copies of written records of consultations to patients, and through the use of 'guided discovery'.

Rather than focusing on changing the patient, GPs can work *with* the patient against a third 'party' – the patient's problem(s). This emphasis on solving problems rather than on a patient's 'defects' reduces any sense of shame, inadequacy or defensiveness and helps patients to work more effectively to bring about change.

To build collaboration, try to use a flexible, negotiating communication style, and avoid playing the role of 'absolute expert'. This involves being open to suggestions, following the patient's lead and being prepared to acknowledge and deal with any misunderstandings or mistakes. It is also important to openly explain all treatment approaches and jointly carry out activities such as writing a problem list or agreeing homework.

Lifting the 'do something' pressure

In a busy surgery, it is common for GPs to feel under pressure to immediately focus on problems and try to solve them as rapidly as possible. GPs may feel that this pressure stems from patients, although it may also arise from their own desire to feel that progress has been made.

In fact, this 'quick-fix' approach is often ineffective because it risks misunderstandings and does not sufficiently engage the patient for any meaningful forward progress to be made. It tends to undermine collaboration by becoming overly didactic and doctor-centred.

Instead, it is more helpful to reduce the pressure for immediate solutions and work collaboratively with patients to understand and agree possible ways of making forward progress through realistic small steps.

From *theory* to *practice*...	You may sometimes notice that you are feeling tense and pressured to try to 'fix' a patient's complex problems in a short time.
	Next time this arises, try to remain aware of this pressure, but not to immediately act on it. As a behavioural experiment, test out some alternative strategies, such as asking the patient to suggest a suitable course of action themselves. If they are not sure, try asking some open questions to help them explore possible options.
	What happens? What are the pros and cons of this approach?

Using guided discovery to build collaboration

Guided discovery involves the joint exploration of problems, where the patient is encouraged to discover key information for themselves, rather than being instructed or led by the clinician. It is analogous to a 'dance' where the GP follows the lead of the patient in discovering what is important to each individual as an expert in their own lives. The GP's role is to support the patient and help them to focus on their most important issues. This involves clarifying, summarising and reflecting back key information.

Socratic questioning is a form of guided discovery where the therapist asks a series of questions to help the patient gain new insight and understanding of their difficulties. For this process, the health professional is not expected to know all the answers and to guide the patient towards these. Instead, it is more helpful to adopt an attitude of curiosity and naivety, and to enjoy the 'journey of discovery' of learning more about the patient, without preconceived ideas and without offering advice or opinions.

Padesky (2003) identified a four-stage process of guided discovery which can be used in CBT sessions (*Box 5.1*).

Expressing empathy

Empathy involves trying to put ourselves in the shoes of another person, and understanding how it might feel to face their particular problems. Empathic statements help to build a strong, trusting relationship between GP and patient.

Box 5.1	**The four stages of guided discovery**

1. Asking informational questions

A series of questions to uncover relevant information outside the patient's current awareness.

2. Empathic listening

Accurate listening and reflection by the therapist.

3. Summarising

Giving summary of information discovered enables patients to consider problems from a new perspective.

4. 'Synthesising' or 'handover' questions

Questions encourage patients to make sense of problems by applying any new information discussed to their original beliefs.

Adapted from Padesky (2003).

Empathy can also be expressed through non-verbal communication such as eye contact, facial expression, nodding when appropriate and encouraging the patient's contribution. Paying attention, picking up on cues and remaining 'present' to the patient's experience also promote effective empathy.

In CBT, the therapist seeks to understand what really matters to a patient, without assuming, guessing or generalising about their experiences. The clinician attempts to "step into the patient's world and see and experience life the way the patient does" (Beck *et al.*, 1979). This is more than simply reassuring patients that they are being heard and understood, but involves attempting to understand the particular thoughts and beliefs that help to explain the patient's reaction (*Box 5.2*).

Box 5.2	**Different types of empathic statement**

General empathic statements

- *"That must be very difficult for you…"*
- *"That sounds really painful…"*
- *"That seems to make you quite angry…"*

Specific empathic statements

- *"It must feel really terrifying if you think 'it must be cancer' every time you get the pain."*
- *"I can understand why you might feel so low when you are having so many negative thoughts about being a failure."*

Being empathic involves understanding how the patient's thinking leads to specific feelings and behaviours, but the clinician *need not agree with the thinking* if it is illogical or exacerbates rather than resolves problems. Nevertheless, it is essential to accept that the patient's thoughts and feelings seem valid to them and should not be dismissed or belittled.

CBT communication skills

One of the most effective ways of beginning to incorporate simple 10 Minute CBT skills into routine practice is to focus on the specific communication or consultation skills (*Box 5.3*) which underpin the approach. The vast majority of GPs are *already* highly practised communicators and, in this way, CBT training simply builds on your existing skills and knowledge.

Box 5.3

Key consultation skills for 10 Minute CBT

1. Problem-focused approach.
2. Identify a specific example of key problems.
3. Explore example using the CBM.
4. Summarise and highlight links between areas of the CBM.
5. Handover (synthesising) questions.
6. Use of empowering explanations.
7. Setting and reviewing homework.
8. Ask for feedback / check patient understanding.

Problem-focused approach

CBT takes a problem-focused approach, where patients are encouraged to break down their problems into manageable 'chunks' and focus on one important area at a time. This often involves setting an 'agenda' for the session by spending a short time agreeing which are the most important issues to discuss in the limited time. This can be therapeutic in its own right, because defining and clarifying problems can make them seem more manageable.

Another strategy is to create a brief problem list with the patient (*Box 5.4*). Patients often have as many as five or more items that they would like to discuss per consultation (Barry *et al.*, 2000), so having an open discussion to prioritise problems can be a helpful way of managing time effectively.

Problem-focused approach: what to say

> *"As we have limited time, I'd like to check what you'd like to discuss today. We may not have time to cover everything but we can come back to anything important next time..."*

Box 5.4

Aims of writing a problem list

- Ensure that all relevant items are covered (or deferred until later).
- Improve collaboration by encouraging the patient to take the lead in planning what to discuss.
- Optimise use of limited time by devoting greater time to most important issues.
- Help patient gain greater clarity about the nature of their problems.

As part of a collaborative partnership, the GP may also wish to add important items onto the problem list for discussion during a particular consultation.

"I also thought it might be helpful to discuss some new ways to cope with your anxiety symptoms..."

Finish by asking the patient to decide which area to focus on first. It can be equally valid to choose the biggest problem, or to pick a difficulty that is less major but may be more easily resolved.

"Which of these areas would be most important for you to focus on today?"

Case Example 5.1: Being problem-focused

John is a 45 year old IT manager who has presented to his GP on several occasions with anxiety and low mood.

GP   "Hello John, how are things?"

John   "Not very good, I'm afraid. I'm really anxious and we are having lots of problems with our son, Andrew. Work is really stressful too."

GP   "That all sounds really difficult. What is the most important problem to talk about today?"

John   "I'm not sure. There are so many things…"

GP   "That's true. But we can make a note of anything we don't cover and come back to it next time. You mentioned that you are concerned about your son and that work is stressful. Should we look at one of these areas today…?"

John   "I think the worst thing is that I am feeling so anxious and low at the moment. It affects every other part of my life."

GP   "Ok, that sounds like a good place to start."

From *theory* to *practice*...

Try collaboratively writing a brief problem list to help plan out one or two of your next consultations. You may wish to choose a patient who often presents with multiple or complex issues. Make sure you do not spend too much of the consultation time setting the agenda itself!

Identify a specific example of key problems

Rather than discussing problems in general terms, ask the patient for a specific and typical example of their problem. This continues to take a problem-focused approach and makes really effective use of the limited consultation time.

Identify a specific example: what to say

Ask for a concrete example of a recent incident that illustrates the problem. Try to identify the details of the incident and when it took place: When, where, who, what, etc.

"Could you give me a recent example of a situation where you felt anxious?"

"When did this take place? Where were you? What were you doing?"

Try to discover at what precise moment the patient experienced a strong negative emotional reaction, and then ask for the negative thoughts which underpinned their reaction.

"At exactly what point did you start to feel bad? What were you doing? At that moment, what was running through your mind?"

Case Example 5.1: *Continued*: choosing a specific example to focus on

The following dialogue continues the discussion between John, a 45 year old IT manager, and his GP.

GP   *"You said that it was most important to discuss the way you are feeling so anxious at the moment?"*

John   *"Yes, I feel anxious so often. I never used to be like this."*

GP   *"That must be very distressing for you. Can you think of an example of a situation in the past week or so when you felt like this?"*

John   *"Yes, lots of times."*

GP   *"It's often useful to focus on one specific incident when you felt bad. Can you think of a recent, 'typical' example?"*

John   *"Err… Yesterday afternoon when I was given a deadline at work to finish a report."*

GP   (Writing the information) *"I see. And at what exact point did you start to feel anxious? What were you doing?"*

John   *"It started as soon as I sat down at my computer to start the report."*

GP   *"That's very helpful. Let's talk about it in a bit more depth…"*

From *theory* to *practice*...

Try asking one or two patients for a specific example of when they experienced a particular problem. How relevant or useful is the information gathered? Can it be generalised to understand the patient as a whole? How does this process affect the flow, amount or type of information generated in the consultation?

Explore the example using the CBM

The next stage is to explore the example and gather information about each of the five areas of the CBM (*Box 5.5*). More details about the key questions to ask about each stage are covered in *Chapter 4*.

Patients often reply to questions with a mixture of information from different areas of the CBM. For example, when asked for feelings, they may reply with thoughts. Rather than correcting the patient, it is more helpful to simply listen carefully and annotate the CBM chart with the relevant information in the appropriate section. When summarising the information back to the patient, try to then break it down correctly into the five areas.

Summarise and highlight links

Summarising is one of the most important CBT skills. People need time and space to make cognitive and emotional changes, and summaries form a natural break in consultations which give the patient an opportunity to reflect.

Summaries can help patients to view their problems from a new perspective, which may be more objective. They also show patients that they have been listened to and that their perspective has been understood.

Try to regularly reflect back the patient's words, highlighting important thoughts, emotions or behaviours:

> "So, when your boss asked to see you, you thought 'I'm going to lose my job. How will I pay the mortgage? We could lose our home', and you started to feel anxious."

> "And when you felt the pain, you thought, 'I'll never get better', and that made you feel very low?"

It is also useful to include some more detailed summaries:

> "I'd like to summarise our discussion so far. You gave me an example of a panic attack last Thursday, when you were about to speak to a group of colleagues. You started feeling anxious and you were thinking: 'What if I have another panic attack? I might make a complete fool of myself.' Physically you noticed that your heart was racing, your hands were sweaty and your chest felt tight.

Then you started thinking, 'It's not normal to feel this bad. Maybe there is something wrong with my heart.' This made you feel even more panicky. You reacted by making an excuse to leave the room and cancelled the meeting. Does that sound accurate?"

Box 5.5	**Summary of useful questions for the CBM**

Thoughts	**Feelings**
"What was going through your mind? What were you thinking?"	*"How did you feel in that situation?"*
"Did you have any images or memories?"	*"When you started to think '………….', how did that make you feel emotionally?"*
"What is most difficult about this for you?"	*"What else were you feeling?"*
"What is the worst that might happen?"	*"You seem quite …..[sad]……. when you say that, is that how you are feeling?"*
Behaviour	**Physical reactions / symptoms**
"What did you do when…? What actions did you take?"	*"How is this affecting you physically?"*
"Are you avoiding any situations because of how you're feeling?"	*"Which symptoms bother you most?"*
"What are you no longer doing now that you feel so depressed / anxious?"	*"How did you feel physically when you were anxious?"*
"What would you do differently if you felt better?"	*"What was happening in your body?"*
Background / environmental factors	
"What else is going on in your life that could be affecting how you feel?"	
"Are there demands at home? Are there financial difficulties?"	
"Do you have someone you can talk to about the problem?"	
"Are there difficulties at work? Are you unable to work / unemployed?"	

Highlighting links

The summary should highlight links between thoughts, feelings or behaviour that have been identified through the discussion. This helps to deepen a patient's understanding of how different aspects of individual problems are connected, and identify potential solutions or areas for change. It is particularly helpful to identify any vicious cycles that are maintaining or worsening problems.

> *"There seems to be a bit of a vicious cycle developing here. When you think negatively you tend to feel low and then react by avoiding seeing people, which makes you feel even more isolated and depressed."*

Handover questions

'Handover' or 'synthesising' questions are a crucial stage of the CBT process, which encourage the patient to reflect and take ownership of making sense of their difficulties (*Box 5.6*). Ask the patient to consider what they can learn or understand from the discussion, and then give them space to reflect on their answer. If the patient hesitates, try not to rush too quickly into offering an answer yourself. Instead, use silence or a second question to encourage the patient to contribute to the discussion.

A summary followed by a handover question is also a very useful approach to take if the consultation has become 'stuck' and you feel uncertain how to proceed. Simply ask the patient what they make of the discussion so far. This is often interesting and enlightening. Being 'stuck' may also indicate that you need to spend more time exploring and understanding the key aspects of the problem.

Box 5.6	**Handover questions**

- *"What do you make of all this…?"*
- *"Does this help you see things any differently?"*
- *"What have you learned / understood from our time together today?"*
- *"What might you say to a friend in the same situation?"*
- *"What do you conclude from our discussion? How could you test those conclusions?"*
- *"Are you surprised by anything you see here?"*

Case Example 5.1: *Continued*: summarising, highlighting links and using handover questions

Let's return to John, the 45 year old IT manager suffering from anxiety and depression. In the previous dialogue, John identified a situation at work where he felt typically stressed and anxious.

Read through the following dialogue and try to identify each of the communication skills that John's GP uses to explore the problem:

GP	*"Imagine yourself back in that situation for a moment. You are sitting at your desk with a report to write. What was going through your mind?"*
John	*"I was thinking 'I'll never get it done on time' and 'It won't be good enough'."*
GP	*"And if it wasn't good enough?"*
John	*"Then I would look like a fool in front of my boss or might even lose my job."*
GP	*"Can you tell me how you were feeling when you were thinking that?"*
John	*"Really anxious."*
GP	*"I see, feeling anxious. Were there any other strong feelings?"*
John	*"I was also feeling sad."*
GP	*"OK, can I check that I understand you? When you sat down at your computer to start the report, you started having some negative thoughts, such as 'I'll never get it done on time', 'It won't be good enough' and 'I will look like a fool in front of my boss and could lose my job'. When you thought those things, you started feeling anxious, sad, tense and sweaty. Does that sound right?"*
John	*"That's exactly how it was."*
GP	*"It sounds very stressful."*
John	*"Yes, it was awful."*
GP	*"Did you have any physical symptoms?"*
John	*"I was feeling tense and sweaty. I started to get a headache."*
GP	*"I see. And how did you react? What did you do?"*
John	*"I just sat there for a while. Then I couldn't face it any more so I started doing something else instead. Eventually I had to do the report but I left it so late that it was a real rush and I don't think it was very good."*
GP	*"I've written down everything you told me. It seems like there may be a bit of a vicious cycle. You said that you were thinking 'I'll never get it done' and 'it won't be good enough' and that made you feel anxious and sad. You reacted by putting off starting the report and then having to rush so it wasn't as good as you would have liked. Tell me, what do you make of all this?"*
John	*"I can see how I've got trapped in a cycle. The more worried I feel about the report, the more I put off starting it, which makes me even more anxious."*
GP	*"Yes, that makes a lot of sense. Now that you have found this vicious cycle, maybe we could look at some ways to turn it into a more positive cycle..."*

<table>
<tr><td>From theory to practice…</td><td>Handover questions are less commonly used in routine GP consultations, so you may need to make a particular effort to adopt this questioning style in your own practice. Try to do so because this is an extremely important step in the CBT process.

After asking a handover question, try to avoid the temptation to jump into the inevitable pause that follows as the patient reflects on their answer! Hold your breath and wait to see what they have to say for themselves.</td></tr>
</table>

Giving empowering explanations

Empowering explanations are important in helping patients to understand and take ownership of both physical and mental health problems, and can be used within any medical consultation (Salmon *et al.*, 1999). Key elements of empowering explanations include:

- open discussions between GP and patient, which acknowledge and legitimise the patient's experiences
- providing tangible causal mechanisms of physical and emotional symptoms
- providing a sense of control over problems and encouraging active self-management (e.g. explanations about 'depression tiredness', see *Chapter 12*)
- discussion of a patient's specific fears, concerns or beliefs about their problems
- encouraging 'exculpation' or removal of any sense of blame or stigma associated with the problems
- building collaboration using interactive dialogue and questions
- avoiding medical jargon.

Giving empowering explanations: what to say

"Would you find it useful to learn a bit more about anxiety and how it can affect the body? What do you know already about anxiety..?"

"Anxiety is very unpleasant but is not actually dangerous. Our anxiety response is designed to help keep us safe from physical dangers. Do you know what happens to the body to do this...?"

"You said that during a panic attack you worry that the chest pain might mean that you are having a heart attack. Perhaps we could talk through some alternative reasons why you might experience chest pain when anxious, which are less serious..."

Setting and reviewing homework

Following up homework

Negotiating actions for the patient to carry out after the session (setting 'homework') is an important stage which enables the patient to apply any new concepts, ideas or CBT principles to their lives. Compliance with homework assignments is a good predictor of the outcome of CBT sessions.

The discussion should also cover any actions for the health professional to carry out, such as making referrals or prescribing medication.

Agreeing homework: what to say

It is important to explain the rationale for homework as well as discussing the reasons for particular tasks.

"Let's think about how to apply what we have talked about today in a practical way to your daily life. The most important thing is what you do differently as a result of the discussion."

Homework tasks should be discussed and planned collaboratively by GP and patient together (*Box 5.7*):

Box 5.7

Setting homework

- *"How could you use this information to make a difference to your life?"*
- *"Now that we've seen the vicious cycle, what could you do differently?"*
- *"If by some miracle, your problems disappeared tomorrow, what would you do differently? Could you do some of those things anyway?"*
- *"What would you do differently if you felt less depressed / more confident / less anxious?"*
- *"Perhaps we could try and 'experiment' to test out what happens...?"*
- *"How might someone else approach this problem? Could you try this?"*

Homework should involve simple, 'SMART' tasks (see *Chapter 8* on goal setting; SMART tasks are Specific, Measurable, Achievable, Relevant and Timely) that are easily achievable by the patient. Some examples of homework tasks are shown in *Box 5.8*.

Homework should be set up as a 'no-lose' experiment. The aim is to try something new and to be open to learning from the result, rather than to achieve any definitive specified outcome.

"I will be very interested to hear how you get on. We can't be certain what will happen, but we can always learn from it, and use it to plan what to try next."

Box 5.8	**Examples of useful homework tasks**

- Taking away a copy of the CBM chart to reflect on and add to further.
- Reading a self-help CBT book or leaflet relevant to their specific difficulties.
- Recording relevant information, such as keeping a diary of thoughts and feelings in different situations.
- Behavioural experiments such as increasing exercise or pleasurable activities, or graded exposure to anxiety-provoking situations.

It is also useful to check that the patient feels able to undertake the homework:

"Are you willing to commit to doing the homework? How confident are you that you could carry it out, on a scale from 1 to 10?"

To remember what was agreed, both GP and patient should keep a *written copy* of the task(s).

Following up homework

Once you have agreed a homework task, it is essential to review and discuss what happened when you next see the patient. Ideally, it should be one of the *first* things to mention when seeing the patient. Otherwise, it sends the message that homework is not really necessary or important and discourages patients from attempting future tasks.

"I am really interested to hear about your homework. What happened …?"

"Did you have a chance to read the leaflet on panic attacks? What did you think about it?"

Overcoming difficulties with homework

There are many reasons why a patient may not complete a homework task. Rather than automatically blaming the patient and assuming that they do not want to change, it is more productive to explore the reasons behind this behaviour. This is a similar principle for patients who do not comply with *any* medical treatment.

Often the reasons that a patient has had difficulty with a homework task mirror the problems they are facing in other areas of their lives. For example, perfectionist patients may become overwhelmed by the amount of effort they perceive would be necessary to produce 'perfect' homework. Patients with procrastination problems may not 'get around' to the homework. Addressing these problems directly will help the patient to understand how their problems affect all aspects of their life, and can help find ways to overcome these issues (*Box 5.9*).

| Box 5.9 | **Overcoming difficulties with homework** |

Reason for not completing homework task	Approach to resolving problem
Patient did not understand the importance of homework.	Discuss why homework is important: *"What could be the benefits of trying this?"* Remind patient that homework predicts likely benefit of CBT, and learning a new skill takes time, effort and practice.
Patient did not understand what they were expected to do.	Remember to check the patient's understanding of homework tasks: *"What are you planning to try this week for your homework?"*
Patient forgot to carry out the task.	Make a written record of homework (e.g. in a journal). Discuss ways to prompt memory: *"How could you remind yourself to try this?"*
Patient did not think homework was useful or relevant.	Design homework in collaboration with the patient: *"Following this discussion, what could you do differently?"* Check understanding of the rationale for homework: *"How might trying this help you...?"*
Lack of time or motivation to carry out the task (seeing homework as a lower priority than other issues).	Try to get explicit agreement and commitment to completing homework. Is the problem important enough to put time and effort into changing? *"How important is it to you to improve your panic attacks?"* Express empathy for the hard work required: *"It can be tough to make changes, especially when life is stressful and busy".*
Task too difficult to carry out (e.g. too anxiety-provoking).	Ensure homework is realistic and achievable: *"How likely do you think you are to be able to do this?"* Discuss possible barriers *before* any potentially difficult or anxiety-provoking task: *"What might get in the way of doing this? How could you get around that?"*

Case Example 5.1: *Continued*: overcoming difficulties with homework

Let's return for a final time to the dialogue between John and his GP. John has returned without having completed the agreed homework – to read through some information about CBT and anxiety.

GP   *"So tell me, how did you find the homework we agreed on last time?"* (Checks written notes.) *"It was to read a leaflet on anxiety, wasn't it? What did you think about it?"*

John   *"Well… I didn't manage to read it."*

GP   *"Oh right. What got in the way of doing it this week?"*

John   *"I just couldn't find the time – I've been really busy at work."*

GP   *"It can be really difficult when you have lots of different pressures to cope with. Tell me, how important is it to you to improve your anxiety? Are you happy to continue as things are?"*

John   *"Oh no, I really want to change. I don't want to feel like this anymore."*

GP   *"Do you think it will be easy to change?"*

John   (Looks demoralised.) *"No, I find it all so difficult. But I don't want to feel like this forever. I'm not sure what to do."*

GP   *"Have you ever learned anything complicated? Can you drive, for example?"*

John   *"Yes, I do drive."*

GP   *"When you were learning to drive, were you able to jump straight into the car and drive perfectly, without any lessons or practice?"*

John   *"No! I had to have quite a few driving lessons."*

GP   *"And what happened to your driving after taking the lessons?"*

John   *"Well, it got better and eventually I passed my test."*

GP   *"But supposing you hadn't made time to practise, do you think you would have improved your driving?"*

John   *"No, I would never have got any better."*

GP   *"Can you see any similarity between learning to drive and trying to learn a new way to cope with your anxiety?"*

John   *"I suppose it is important to keep practising otherwise I will never get any better."*

GP   *"Yes, that seems true to me too. And how does homework fit in with all this? What is the purpose of it?"*

John   *"It is a way to practise and to get over my anxiety. It is important to me, so I will try harder to make some time for this."*

From *theory* to *practice*...	Remember to remain collaborative when setting homework tasks. If you notice the patient is not contributing ideas, or is saying 'yes, but...' it may be that you are being overly didactic in setting homework *for* the patient rather than *with* the patient. Instead, try asking the patient for their own thoughts and suggestions.

Ask for feedback / check patient understanding

The final step is to ask the patient for feedback about the consultation. This strengthens relationships with patients and increases their involvement in the consultation.

"I would like you to let me know if anything does not make sense or if I misunderstand you. This will help us to work together most effectively."

Asking for feedback also enables the GP to check the patient's perspective of the CBT approach.

"How have you found this approach? Does it all make sense to you?"

Checking a patient's understanding of what has been discussed is also essential for clarifying information and preventing misunderstandings. This is particularly important in conditions such as health anxiety, where doctor–patient misunderstandings are common and may significantly worsen the patient's problems (see *Chapter 15*).

"I'd just like to check what you will take away from our discussion today. What were the most important things that we talked about?"

Key learning points

- Learning specific communication and consultation skills offers a practical way of bringing a brief CBT approach into routine practice.
- Try to encourage the patient to engage and contribute to the session, as this will help to build a strong relationship that facilitates positive change.
- Use guided discovery to work with the patient to understand problems, set goals and work on solutions.
- Be aware that you may sometimes feel a pressure to fix the patient's problem, but that it is usually more effective to step back and allow the patient to take the lead.

Communication skill	Remember	What to say
Problem-focused approach	Try setting a brief agenda or creating a problem list at the start of consultations, to help optimise the use of limited time. Allow the patient to prioritise their most important issues.	*"Let's plan how we will use our limited time today..."* *"Let's make a list of your main problems..."* *"What is the most important thing you'd like to discuss today?"*
Identify a specific example of key problems	Ask for specific, recent examples of incidents which illustrate the patient's problem(s).	*"Can you give me a recent example of this problem?"* *"When was this? Where were you? What were you doing at the time?"*
Explore example using the CBM	Discuss the example in depth using the CBM as a guide. Remember to make empathic statements based on the particular thoughts, feelings and behaviours that contribute towards a patient's distress.	*"What was going through your mind?"* *"How were you feeling?"* *"Any physical symptoms?"* *"What did you do?"* *"What else is going on at the moment?"*
Summarise and highlight links between areas of the CBM	Make frequent summaries and reflective statements, particularly if you are feeling a bit 'stuck' and unsure of where to go next. Use the patient's own words and point out any links between areas of the CBM or vicious cycles.	*"This is what I've heard you tell me today..."* *"I noticed that when you started to think negatively, you also started to feel quite low..."*
Handover (synthesising) questions	Use handover questions to encourage the patient to make sense of the information and learn from it themselves.	*"What do you make of what we have discussed today?"* *"Is there anything you might learn from this?"*

Communication skill	Remember	What to say
Use of empowering explanations	Provide positive, tangible explanations of problems which give patients a sense of control over their difficulties. Include any specific thoughts or fears that the patient holds in the explanation.	*"I'd like to give another, less serious, explanation of your chest pain. I know you are worried that it may be your heart, but I believe the pain is coming from the muscles in your chest wall"*
Setting and reviewing homework	Homework may involve reflecting on key information or testing out new behaviours and approaches to difficulties. Tasks should be 'SMART' and agreed collaboratively by GP and patient. Always discuss what happened during the next appointment.	*"What would you like to try out after this discussion?"* *"What small step could you take towards your goal?"* *"How confident are you that you could achieve this? Do we need to make this goal more realistic?"*
Ask for feedback/ check patient understanding	Ask for feedback on the patient's experience of the consultation and the CBT approach. You must be flexible and willing to revise your opinion when necessary, and to correct any misunderstandings that may have arisen.	*"How did you find this session today?"* *"What will you take away from our discussion?"*

Chapter 6

Coping with negative thoughts

How can changing thoughts help?

Finding new perspectives for difficult situations can alter the vicious cycles that contribute to the development and maintenance of mood disorders and emotional distress.

This chapter will outline some core cognitive change methods, which represent an important aspect of the CBT approach, and suggest some ways of using them in a GP consultation. However, it is important to recognise that it can be difficult to implement complex thought-changing strategies in a collaborative way during a brief consultation. Other approaches such as behaviour change (*Chapter 7*) may be more effective in this setting.

Unhelpful thinking styles

Some negative ways of looking at the world can become a pattern or habitual way of thinking – these are known as unhelpful thinking styles (*Box 6.1*) and represent distorted or skewed ways of viewing the world. Identifying unhelpful thinking patterns provides the first step towards balanced thinking and improved moods.

To avoid patients feeling guilty or foolish for having unhelpful thoughts, you can explain that unhelpful thinking styles are common and everyone uses them sometimes. Nevertheless, looking for an alternative view may help people to feel better.

From *theory* to *practice*... Give patients a written information leaflet about unhelpful thinking styles to read at home. Suggest that they try to pick out their own typical unhelpful thinking styles and then keep a diary noticing how often these thoughts arise.

Can they think of any alternative ways to look at the situation using the prompts in the leaflet?

Box 6.1	Unhelpful thinking styles
All or nothing (black and white) thinking	Viewing things in 'all or nothing' terms without taking into account any possibilities between the two extremes, e.g. *"Nobody likes me. I am a total failure".* **Shades of grey** It is rare for anything to be either 100% perfect or a complete disaster. Try to be realistic and take into account both positive and negative events. Use a 'positive diary' to remind you of any achievements or good moments.
Catastrophic thinking	Jumping to extreme conclusions when something goes wrong and predicting dire consequences in the future, e.g. *"I made a mistake at work so I'll probably lose my job".* **Keep a realistic view of the future** Try to keep a balanced view without jumping to the worst conclusion. Focus on the here and now and what you can do to solve the problems that you are facing.
"What if...?" statements	Constantly worrying about future problems and disasters without planning how to cope with these difficulties, e.g. *"What if I panic when I get to the shops...? What if he thinks I'm stupid...?"* **The worst may not happen!** Focus on how you might cope if things do go wrong – *"Then what would I do to cope...?"* Write your solutions down.
Emotional reasoning	Acting as if subjective feelings are concrete facts, e.g. *"I feel unattractive so I must be. I feel so anxious thinking about going to the shops, I'll never be able to cope when I get there".* **Your emotions may be clouding your judgement** When emotions are running high we tend to think in more extreme and exaggerated ways. Take a deep breath and make decisions when feeling calmer. Try asking for feedback or 'reality checks' from others.

Box 6.1 Continued	Blaming yourself (taking too much personal responsibility)	Unfairly seeing yourself as the cause of bad events, even when you are not really to blame, e.g. *"It's my fault that my partner cheated on me".* **Share the responsibility fairly** You are not the only person who is responsible for problems. Try making a list of everyone involved in a particular situation, including yourself only at the end. You might discover that, although you do have some responsibility, *it is not entirely your fault.*
	Self-criticism (and name calling)	Tending to be overly critical and negative about yourself, you may also call yourself by harsh or unkind names, e.g. *"I always mess everything up. I can't do this – I'm so stupid!"* **Be kind and compassionate to yourself and others** Don't ignore your achievements in life – both small and large. It's impossible for anyone to mess *everything* up! Would you be as harsh on your best friend? If not, remember it's only fair to use the same rules for ourselves as for others.
	Mind reading (negative view about how others see you)	Assuming that others think the worst about you, e.g. *"He thinks I'm such a loser".* **Don't jump to the worst conclusion!** Others may not be thinking the worst. People are often more concerned with their own problems than with what you have said or done. Keep in mind the positive opinions of those who like and care about you.
	Ignoring the positive	Ignoring, dismissing or rejecting any positive events or messages, e.g. *"He's only saying that because he feels sorry for me. That was nothing special – anyone could do that".* **Remember life is made up of positives and negatives** Try to keep in mind both positives and negatives and allow yourself to acknowledge your successes rather than simply dwelling on problems.

Box 6.1 Continued	**Unrealistic high standards**	Being a perfectionist and setting standards that are impossible to achieve. Using 'should', 'ought to' and 'must' statements, e.g. *"I should never make a mistake. I must be liked by everyone".*
		Be more flexible and realistic about your goals
		Switch 'should' to 'would prefer...', e.g. *"I would like to always say the best thing, but no one can be perfect, so I will just do my best".*

The problem with trying not to think negatively

Many people instinctively try to suppress or control unpleasant negative automatic thoughts, e.g. *"I just try to ignore or block out my worries".* Unfortunately, this is not a very effective strategy for reducing the power or frequency of negative thoughts in the long term (see *Box 6.2*).

Box 6.2	**Pink elephant experiment**
	For the next 30 seconds, try as hard as you can *not to* think about a pink elephant.
	What happened? Did you think about the pink elephant at all? Was this easy or did it take a lot of mental effort?
	Many people find that thoughts and images of the elephant pop into the mind despite efforts to keep them out. Trying *not to* think about a particular thought takes a great deal of mental effort and often has a converse effect of making the thought even more prominent.
	Imagine how much more difficult this exercise would be for someone trying to suppress terrifying images about a particular feared situation.

Trying to ignore or suppress negative thoughts may paradoxically *increase* their power. In trying *not to* think something, the unpleasant thought or image is likely to flash into the mind, where it triggers distressing emotions.

A more effective method of dealing with unhelpful thoughts is to accept their presence, identify what they are and then find ways to actively challenge and reframe them.

Distraction

Distraction is a useful short-term method of managing negative thoughts by paying attention to something else. It is particularly helpful for anxiety disorders, and may also be useful for depression when people are becoming overwhelmed by large numbers of negative thoughts throughout the day.

Distraction is not a long-term solution that challenges negative thoughts or helps patients think more rationally. However, it does offer a simple, rapid, 'first-aid' strategy to reduce the power of negative thinking, by taking the patient's mind away from distressing or unhelpful thoughts. This can reduce powerful negative feelings to more manageable levels, when it becomes easier to see problems from a more rational perspective.

Distraction differs from attempting to simply suppress or ignore negative thoughts because it involves a positive rather than a negative command for the mind. It involves trying to actively engage in a particular activity, which has the additional benefit of taking the mind away from negative thoughts.

The best distraction activities are able to fully engage the mind, but are not too complex or difficult. Help the patient to plan in advance which distraction technique they will try in particular difficult situations, and then to monitor what effect it had (*Box 6.3*).

Box 6.3

Useful distraction techniques

- Do simple puzzles such as crosswords, word searches, jigsaws.
- Search the internet, play a musical instrument or a computer game.
- Raise activity levels: go for a walk, follow a yoga DVD, do a household job.
- Perform simple mental arithmetic (e.g. take 7 away from 100 and repeat).
- Copy or draw a diagram or picture.
- Count objects, e.g. number of bricks in a wall, number of colours or hues in a picture.
- Mentally describe what you can see, hear, smell or feel out of the window.

Difficulties with using distraction

There is a risk that patients use distraction as a 'safety behaviour' to avoid *ever* facing problems or overcoming negative thoughts and beliefs. In this case, distraction can be counterproductive and simply serves as an avoidance tactic. Encourage the patient to use distraction as only the *first step* in managing unpleasant thoughts and emotions. The next step is to face up to and make changes to negative thoughts.

From *theory* to *practice*...

Distraction is a quick strategy which can be demonstrated during a consultation for an anxious patient. Ask the patient to rate their anxiety from 0 to 100 (where 0 is no anxiety at all and 100 is the most anxious they could possibly imagine).

Then ask the patient to describe an object in the room or out of the window in great detail. You can prompt with questions about colour, shape, size, smell, etc. Try to ask questions that make the patient *think* about the object (e.g. *"What else could you use this for?"* or *"What might the person outside the window be doing or thinking about?"*).

After 1–2 minutes, ask the patient to re-rate their level of anxiety. If it remains high, repeat the experiment with a different form of distraction. For example, ask the patient to copy or draw around a geometrical shape on a piece of paper.

Once the patient's anxiety has decreased, try to use this as a learning experience by asking:

"How do you feel now? What do you make of the fact that you can feel better so quickly?"

"How could you use this to help you in the future?"

"What was going through your mind that made you feel so anxious? Do you see things any differently now you feel calmer?"

Broadening perspectives on difficult situations

It can be helpful to encourage the patient to put difficult situations into perspective. How serious a mistake was it *really?* How important is this problem in the bigger scheme of things?

One way of gaining perspective on problems is to ask patients to imagine how they might view the event in the future.

"How will you feel about this in a year's time? Will it still be as important then?"

"How about in 5 years' time? What about in 10 years...?"

Pie charts can also be a useful tool for exploring alternative explanations for events. The aim is to generate a more balanced view, by looking at a range of factors which may be involved. This can lessen the fear of any particularly negative or catastrophic outcome. Pie charts are useful in anxiety disorders, where people tend to overestimate the risk of potential future events, and can also be used to evaluate feelings of excessive responsibility or guilt after a difficult experience. An example of using a pie chart in health anxiety is given in *Chapter 15*.

Another useful technique to gain perspective is to use a 'severity scale', where the patient compares different events on a scale from extremely serious to unimportant (see *Case Example 6.1*).

Case Example 6.1: Using a 'severity scale' to gain perspective

Paula is a 35 year old secretary. As she arrives at the annual office party, she trips over in front of her boss. She is not hurt and gets up quickly, but for many weeks afterwards, Paula worries about the incident and feels increasingly anxious and low. She even begins taking time off work to avoid facing her colleagues.

Thoughts:

"It was such a stupid thing to do."   "Everyone was laughing at me."

"I looked like a complete fool."

Paula's GP suggests that she could make a list of other problems that could arise at an office party. This included some very unlikely or humorous possibilities, for example:

- get angry and throw a drink over an important client
- accidentally smash a valuable antique vase
- get drunk and vomit onto the carpet
- get caught stealing money from colleagues
- start a fight and get arrested
- start a fire and burn the restaurant down

Paula's GP asks her to rate these possibilities into order of severity, using a 'severity scale'. Only after including all the other possibilities does she add the actual 'mistake' that she had made onto the scale:

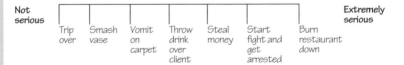

Not serious								Extremely serious
	Trip over	Smash vase	Vomit on carpet	Throw drink over client	Steal money	Start fight and get arrested	Burn restaurant down	

This exercise helps put the severity or importance of Paula's experience into perspective and helps to illustrate that her negative thoughts about tripping over were extreme and unfair.

Useful questions to encourage patients to reflect on this exercise include:

"What do you make of this? Does this give you any different perspective on what happened?"

Evaluating negative thoughts

Identifying negative thoughts

The first step is to teach people to notice and identify their thoughts which are leading to particular emotional reactions. The aim is to identify the most relevant or 'hot' thought (Greenberger & Padesky, 1995a), that is usually associated with the most powerful feelings of emotional distress.

It is helpful to write thoughts down, using a diary or written thought record. This makes the thoughts seem more 'concrete', easier to clarify and helps people to view them from a more rational perspective.

Evaluating the evidence for thoughts

Evaluating the evidence for particular thoughts involves exploring the reasons why the patient holds a particular negative belief, without initially challenging or attempting to change it.

The next step is to look for any evidence that suggests the thought may *not* be entirely accurate. This includes considering whether the thought is logical, realistic or represents an unhelpful thinking style (see *Box 6.4*). Finally, the patient is encouraged to take all the evidence into account, both positive and negative, in order to come up with a more balanced and realistic perspective.

Box 6.4

Questions to evaluate the evidence for negative thoughts

- What is the evidence for this thought? What makes you think that?
- Is there any evidence against this thought? Does anything suggest it might not be entirely accurate?
- Is it logical or realistic? Is it fair?
- Is it a compassionate or kind way of looking at things?
- Is it an 'unhelpful' thinking style?
- What are the advantages and disadvantages of thinking this way?
- What advice would you give to someone else in this situation?
- Is there another way to view the situation that takes all of this new evidence into account?

Using written thought records

Written thought records provide a structured way of identifying and evaluating negative thoughts and beliefs. The patient should write down how they thought and felt during a difficult situation or at a time of emotional distress. To remember this information clearly, it is helpful to fill in a thought record as soon as possible after a difficult situation.

Regularly completing thought records will begin to improve a patient's ability to think in more flexible and helpful ways and reduce unhelpful, distorted thinking styles. Eventually, automatic, balanced thoughts may begin to arise automatically in the mind, without the need to complete a written thought record. This may result in patients feeling less distressed in situations that would previously have triggered painful, negative feelings.

The patient can use a thought record like a diary, to record information about:
- situation: what happened, where was it, who was involved, at what point did the patient begin to feel emotionally distressed?
- feelings (rated 0–100)
- thoughts associated with the negative feelings
- the most powerful or distressing thought ('hot' thought).

From *theory* to *practice*...

Tips for completing thought records.

- Write down thoughts using the patient's own words and in the first person (*"He thinks I'm boring"*).
- Be specific about thoughts – find out what the patient actually means by *"It will be terrible"*. How will it be terrible? What might happen? What images do they have?
- If thoughts are expressed as a question then sensitively ask questions that help the patient to reword it as a statement, such as: *"What is your biggest fear? What might go wrong?"*). For example, the thought, *"Will I be able to cope at the cinema?"* can be reworded as *"I won't cope at the cinema, I'll have a panic attack and have to leave"*).

Case Example 6.2: Learning to use a thought record

Sanjay is a 35 year old man who works as a planning officer for a local council. About 3 months ago he was promoted to a senior managerial position that involves giving presentations to other colleagues in the council. He has become increasingly anxious about public speaking and is beginning to avoid these situations, which makes it difficult for him to do his job. He completes a thought record as follows.

Section of thought record	Useful questions	Answers by Sanjay
Situation	*"Describe a typical situation when you felt upset or emotional"* *"At what point did you feel the worst? What were you doing?"*	*"On Thursday at 11 a.m. My boss came into my office and asked me to give a presentation about changes in local planning policy to the heads of department in the council"*

Feelings	"Make a list of all your feelings or emotions" "Rate how strong each feeling was from 0–100 (where 0 is no emotion and 100 is the strongest feeling you could ever imagine)"	"Anxious – 75" "Tense – 70" "Low – 60"
Thoughts	"What went through your mind that made you feel that way?" "What thoughts or images did you have?" "What is the worst bit about this situation?" "What does this situation say about you, your life or your future?" "Are you afraid that something might happen? What is this?" "What might someone else think or feel about you? What does this mean to you?"	"I don't have enough authority or experience and they won't respect me" "I might get so nervous that I can't speak properly and won't be able to get my point across" "I might not know enough about the subject" "What if they don't agree with me or ask me questions that I can't answer?" "They will think I am foolish and incompetent"
Find the hot thought	"Which of these thoughts is the most upsetting?"	**"They will think I am foolish and incompetent"**

Challenging unhelpful thoughts using written thought records

Once the hot thought is identified, it is then possible to challenge its accuracy. As usual, this first involves gathering any detailed evidence that supports and explains why the patient holds this belief, followed by any evidence that does not support the belief.

Thought: "*I am boring*"
Evidence 'for' this belief: "*I don't have much to say to people at work*"
Evidence 'against': "*My friend Liz often calls me up for a chat and we have plenty to talk about*"

The final stage is to generate a new, more balanced thought to replace the original one. This takes into account the evidence both for and against the negative thought. For example:

"*I am quiet in some situations but I have many friends who find me interesting and enjoy my company*"

It is important that this alternative thought is backed up by genuine evidence from the patient's life, so that it seems believable and realistic. This process can be associated with a marked improvement in mood.

Case Example 6.2: *Continued*: **learning to use thought records**

Let's return to Sanjay's thought record, about his anxiety relating to making presentations to colleagues.

Hot thought to test out:	
"They will think I am incompetent and foolish"	
Evidence *for* hot thought:	**Evidence *against* the 'hot' thought:**
What makes you say that this thought is true? Has anything happened to prove it to you? Do any past experiences fit this belief?	Is there anything that shows this thought is not always true? Are there any times when you think differently to this? When? In 5 or 10 years from now, would you look back on this situation any differently? Are you ignoring any positives in the situation? Is this way of thinking an 'unhelpful' thinking style? What would be more realistic or helpful? If your best friend had this thought, what would you tell them?
"Many of the people in the audience have worked for the council a lot longer than I have" "If I seem nervous then people will assume that I don't have much knowledge" "Last week a colleague made a comment about how young I am" "In my last presentation, I was asked a question that I could not answer and became very flustered"	"I have got the qualifications to do my job – that's why I was appointed" "My boss seems confident that I can do it" "I have more training in this area than anyone in the audience" "At the end of my last presentation, another colleague said it was interesting" "I have seen another presenter who could not answer a question from the audience. He just offered to find out after the session" "There are many other parts of my work that I do well. These things also affect how colleagues view me"

> **Alternative / balanced thought to replace the hot thought:**
> Write an alternative or balanced thought which takes into account evidence for and against the hot thought. Try to be fair and realistic.
> *"I am qualified to give this presentation because I am more of an expert in planning than many others in the council. If I don't know the answer to a question I could look up the information afterwards"*
>
> **Rate moods / emotions again** *How do you feel now? Is this any different to before?*
> *Anxious – 40, Tense – 30, Low – 20.*

Overcoming difficulties with thought records

If, after completing a thought record, a patient does not feel an improvement in mood, it can be helpful to use the following checklist of questions:

- Was the situation that was described specific enough? Did the patient focus on the key moment of emotional change?
- Did the patient identify the 'hottest' thought? Are there other key thoughts that are generating the patient's negative feelings?
- Was the thought being tested directly related to the specific feeling that the patient was trying to improve?
- Did the patient write down enough evidence 'against' the hot thought? Did this include alternative ways to view any evidence 'for' the negative thought?
- Does the balanced, alternative thought seem believable and realistic to the patient?
- Does the hot thought actually represent a core belief or a 'rule for living'? These are more deeply held beliefs which may not be effectively altered using a thought record (see *Chapter 10*).

Key learning points

- Learning to think more flexibly, rationally and compassionately can help to reduce emotional distress.
- Start by simply encouraging the patient to identify their thoughts. Remember this can be distressing for the patient if the thoughts are negative or anxiety-provoking.
- Be curious. Take time to explore and understand why the patient holds a negative thought before encouraging them to make any changes.
- The goal is to create an alternative, balanced thought, which takes into account both positive and negative factors. The alternative thought must seem credible and believable or there will be no emotional shift.

Useful strategies for managing negative thoughts and encouraging a more balanced perspective include the following.

- Use simple distraction techniques to keep the mind occupied, such as drawing, looking on the internet or going for a walk. Make sure the distraction strategy does not become a 'prop' or safety behaviour.
- Use a severity scale to put minor problems into perspective; use humour and be creative when trying this approach.
- Imagine how you might view the same situation in 5 or 10 years' time.
- Use a diary to record thoughts that arise in challenging situations, filling it out as soon as possible after the event.
- A written thought record provides a structured way of identifying and reframing negative thoughts. However, this is time-consuming and difficult to complete within a very brief consultation. The patient may need to practise at home using a CBT-based self-help book or work with a CBT therapist to learn to use this effectively.

Chapter 7

Changing unhelpful behaviour

The importance of changing behaviour

Changing behaviour can be one of the most powerful methods of breaking vicious cycles and creating lasting change in difficult emotions. Behavioural change provides powerful *evidence* for changes in thoughts or beliefs. Behavioural experiments give patients the opportunity to test out new beliefs and approaches to problems in real life, which will make them seem more credible and believable.

It is helpful to combine both cognitive and behavioural change. For example, the belief "*I am boring and people don't want to hear my views*" can be discussed and reframed on a verbal or intellectual basis, to a new, more rational perspective such as "*Many people do find my conversation interesting*". However, without also changing the behaviour that is associated with the belief (e.g. avoiding social contact, making poor eye contact with others, not speaking in the company of others), the belief in the new perspective is likely to remain limited. By changing behaviour (e.g. acting 'as if' I am interesting, making eye contact and listening to others, and trying out making conversation), and noting the impact of the change, the patient gathers evidence to reinforce the new, more helpful belief ("*If I do talk to others then they often seem interested in what I have to say*").

Involving patients in behavioural changes

Patients must be actively involved in the cognitive behavioural approach and should be encouraged to take responsibility for making behavioural changes. Health professionals should try to avoid offering excessive advice or solutions which may not be realistic or appropriate within an individual patient's life. Most patients are more likely to follow through ideas they have generated themselves, rather than advice given by others.

'Yes, but...' responses are a common indicator that a health professional's suggestions are too prescribed or directive. Patients may say this directly (e.g. "*Well, yes, I know I should exercise more, but I just don't have time*"), or may outwardly agree, but simply ignore the suggestion once they leave the surgery. This lack of 'concordance' is often seen when prescribing medication.

To avoid 'yes, but...' responses, the simple answer is to make fewer suggestions. Instead, *hand over responsibility to the patient* to generate their own suggestions and choices about realistic, appropriate or useful changes in behaviour.

> *"What do you think might help you in this situation...?"*

> *"You are an 'expert' in your own life. What do you think might work for you?"*

> *"What do you think you could do differently...?"*

Setting realistic expectations for improvement

The process of making behavioural changes should be broken up into small, manageable steps. These are easier to achieve and provide a building block for further change. Patients can be encouraged to carry out a variety of simple experiments to look at different aspects of their difficulties.

Remind patients that making change is not always easy. It is helpful to expect difficulties and to plan ways to actively face and overcome any problems that may arise, rather than simply giving up when things do not immediately go according to plan.

From *theory* to *practice...*

Encourage patients to have realistic expectations about their progress by drawing out a series of boxes, joined by arrows:

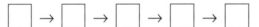

Tell the patient that the box at the far left represents how they are at the current time – ask the patient to describe briefly what this means to them, e.g. *feeling very depressed, not going out, not working.*

The box at the far right represents where they would *like to get to*, e.g. *no longer depressed, back at work, good social life.*

Next, ask the patient to imagine how they might feel in the series of boxes in between:

Still quite low, going out a little more but not really enjoying it, not yet back at work

↓

Mood lifts at times, more active generally, thinking about work

↓

Depression improving, still down occasionally, better social life, preparing to return to work

This helps set realistic targets. It may also be helpful for the patient to realise that it is normal to continue to experience some unpleasant symptoms, even whilst life is improving.

Behavioural activation

Behavioural activation (BA) has been shown to be as effective as antidepressants and possibly even more effective than standard CBT for the management of depression (Dimidjian *et al.*, 2006).

BA is based on the principle that depressed individuals typically behave differently and engage less frequently in enjoyable or satisfying activities. This depressed behaviour is viewed as a form of avoidance, which reinforces depression as a vicious cycle, leading to a lower mood and even more depressed behaviour.

BA involves activity scheduling to encourage depressed people to increase enjoyable and meaningful activities, despite negative feelings or a lack of motivation. This includes planning particular activities that a patient is currently avoiding as well as setting goals that are in line with an individual's valued life directions, such as a return to work and social roles.

It also involves evaluating the underlying thoughts and beliefs that are getting in the way of increased activity. For example:

"I will be more active when I feel better or feel more motivated"

"I can't be bothered – I'm too tired"

"I won't enjoy it anyway"

In contrast to standard CBT, BA places less emphasis on evaluating or debating negative thoughts. Instead, patients are taught to distance themselves from thoughts in a similar process to mindfulness (see *Chapter 11*). The aim is for the patient to acknowledge negative thoughts, but to learn to distance themself from them so that they no longer engage with or 'buy into' them.

The patient is encouraged to plan their behaviour according to the activity schedule, rather than according to how they think or feel at the time. Waiting longer to start a particular activity is likely to make them feel even less motivated. 'Just doing it' or behaving 'as if' they feel better will gradually increase motivation, improve mood and self-esteem.

BA is covered further in *Chapter 12* on depression.

Using 'behavioural experiments'

Behavioural experiments are specifically designed approaches to changing behaviour which are often used in CBT. They allow people to test negative beliefs or predictions and to construct and test new, more adaptive perspectives. Provided the patient remains open to the possibility that an alternative belief *might* have some validity, it is not necessary for them to fully believe it in order to test negative and alternative beliefs. This approach is useful for 'yes, but...' responses. Instead of offering the answer, encourage the patient to *find out for themselves*, by trying out their belief in practice.

Behavioural experiments can be used to collect data that support the development of more positive or helpful beliefs. This is important if the patient simply does not have enough factual material to decide whether or not a particular negative thought is true. For example, people who suffer from social anxiety may hold a belief that *it is abnormal to feel anxious when meeting others – it means there is something wrong with me*. It is only by testing out this belief in practice, perhaps by conducting a small survey of other people's experiences, that patients are able to convincingly establish a new belief such as, *it is common to feel anxious when meeting others*.

Behavioural experiments can also be used to find methods of reducing unpleasant emotional experiences, such as by testing out the impact of using distraction techniques or of using gentle exercise to increase energy in depression.

Identifying relevant behavioural experiments

In order to be effective, behavioural experiments must be directly relevant to individual patients and should test the specific negative, unhelpful beliefs that maintain their problems. It is therefore essential to spend some time developing a thorough understanding of the patient's problems first.

Behavioural experiments can be *active*, where the patient tries out something different and notes down the impact of the new behaviour. Other experiments may be simply *observational*, which might involve asking a patient to observe other people in order to identify new ways of behaving in target situations (which can later be tested out during a more active experiment). It may also be useful for patients to gather a range of information or opinions from other people about particular questions or concerns.

Designing and implementing effective behavioural experiments

There are four systematic steps for designing an effective behavioural experiment and these are outlined in *Box 7.1* and then subsequently described in more detail in the text (see also *Figure 7.1*).

Box 7.1	**Stages for planning behavioural experiments**

1. **Identify the problem** including relevant thoughts, negative predictions, feelings and existing behaviour.
2. **Plan changes to test out** using a detailed, 'no-lose' plan which is realistic and acceptable to the patient and is relevant to the key negative beliefs being tested.
3. **Try out the new behaviour** and keep a written record of what happened.
4. **Review and reflect** on what the information means to the patient and how it can be used to improve life. This includes problem-solving to overcome any difficulties and planning relevant future experiments.

Thought being tested:	
What am I going to do? (what, where, when…?)	
What do I predict will happen?	
What problems might arise with this plan?	
How could these problems be overcome?	
What happened when I tried the experiment?	
What have I learned from this experiment?	

Figure 7.1: Behavioural experiment planning chart

1. Identify the problem

This involves identifying the patient's current behavioural strategies for dealing with their difficulties, in addition to any relevant thoughts, fears or negative predictions about making change.

It is important to be concrete and specific when identifying particular thoughts and negative predictions to test. For example, a socially anxious patient may believe, *I will look foolish in front of others*, but this should be discussed in more depth to identify in what precise ways they fear 'looking foolish', such as *I will babble uncontrollably* or *My mind will go blank and I will say nothing at all.*

The next stage is to identify which behaviours could be altered or changed in order to challenge the underlying negative thoughts. Try to identify a specific, testable prediction based on the patient's thoughts. This involves identifying what the patient thinks will be the consequences of changing the behaviour.

Case Example 7.1: Improving sleep patterns

Trisha is 28 years old and has been depressed for over a year. She is a single mother with a 4 year old daughter. She feels constantly exhausted and lethargic, but sleeps poorly at night – she finds it difficult to drop off to sleep and tends to oversleep in the morning. She has begun taking daytime naps to try to compensate for this.

Her GP helps Trisha to plan out a behavioural experiment to test out the effect of changing her behaviour:

Key thought(s) to test:	I need to take naps to catch up on my lost sleep otherwise I can't cope during the day
	Taking naps makes me feel better when I'm down.
What negative emotions are associated with these thoughts?	Lethargy, feeling down
What current behaviours are reinforcing negative thoughts?	Oversleeping in mornings may make sleep at night worse
What does the patient predict will happen?	I will feel more tired if I don't take a nap.
	My mood will get worse if I'm more tired.
What could be a more balanced and rational belief?	Taking naps makes me feel more tired and low.
	If I stop taking naps, I will still be able to cope and will sleep better at night.

---

2. Plan behavioural changes

The next stage is to decide what behaviour to change in order to test the relevant thoughts. This involves working out a detailed plan of how to conduct the experiment, which includes anticipating and preparing for any difficulties that might arise (*Box 7.2*).

Experiments should be planned as 'no-lose' experiences. This means keeping a genuinely open mind about what might arise. Some apparently unrealistic negative thoughts may turn out to be true. However, discovering this is still useful, because it enables the patient to then focus on effective problem-solving to find a way to overcome it.

The experiments chosen should be relevant, realistic and acceptable to the patient but should not be overly complex or challenging. The GP must be supportive and openly acknowledge the difficulty of trying out something different. This helps the patient face potentially difficult or frightening situations.

Remember to convey enthusiasm and interest in the experiment and its results to the patient, which might encourage them to carry it out.

Box 7.2

Checklist for planning behavioural changes

Planning what experiment to try

- How could you test out whether the key thought is true?
- What could you try doing differently?

Planning how to go about the experiment

- What are the details of the plan (what, when, where, who….)?
- How can we ensure that this is a 'no-lose' experiment?

Preparing for potential difficulties with the experiment

- *"Do you understand what you are trying to do and why?"*
- *"How likely are you to try it? Would anything make you more likely to do so?"*
- *"What problems might arise with trying this? How could you overcome these?"*

Case Example 7.1: *Continued*: improving sleep patterns

Let's return to the example of Trisha, who has identified the following alternative thought to test out: *If I stop taking naps, I will still be able to cope and will sleep better at night.*

Trisha and her GP agree that a helpful way to test this thought would be to compare the two strategies (napping versus not napping) over a two week period. During the first week, Trisha planned not to make any changes to her current sleep pattern, but would monitor how often she napped, how much sleep she got at night and how tired she felt during the day. During the second week, she would try to avoid napping. She would continue to monitor her tiredness and sleep at night. Potential difficulties were that she might feel so tired that she was unable to avoid dropping off to sleep. To try to overcome this problem, Trisha planned some enjoyable activities to try at these times instead.

3. Try out new behaviour and observe what happened

The next step is for the patient to try out the new behaviour in practice. They should be encouraged to keep a written record of what they tried and what happened, in terms of changes in thoughts, feelings or physical symptoms (see *Box 7.3*). In some cases, it may also be necessary to note the reactions of other people.

Box 7.3

Checklist for assessing the outcome of making behavioural changes

- What did you actually do? Was this what you had planned? If not, what got in the way?
- What thoughts arose in your mind before, during and after the experiment?
- How did you *feel*, before, during and after the experiment?
- Did you experience any changes in physical symptoms?
- What did you notice about other people's reactions?

Case Example 7.1: *Continued*: improving sleep patterns

Trisha returned to visit her GP three weeks after the experiment had been carried out.

She found that it had been difficult to reduce her daytime naps, but she had successfully managed to reduce the number of naps from 11 in the first week down to 3 in the second week.

She noticed that at the start of the week it was more difficult to avoid napping and she did feel more tired, but she had still managed to cope with daily life. By the end of the week, she found it easier and felt less lethargic and tired than previously. She also noticed that she was sleeping better at night and that her overall mood had improved.

---

4. Review and reflection

The final stage is for patients to review the results of the experiment and reflect on what it means for them (*Box 7.4*). This is essential for making sense of the information and learning from the experiment.

It is also important to reflect on any difficulties that arose during the experiment and look for ways to move forwards using this information. This may mean trying another experiment to test out another relevant belief. Sometimes patients may try a behaviour which does not help them or a feared prediction may come true. In this case, it is important to encourage patients to creatively *problem-solve* rather than just give up entirely.

Box 7.4

Questions for reviewing and reflecting on behavioural experiments

Learning from the experience

- *"What do you make of what happened?"*
- *"Does this alter your view of your original, negative thought or prediction?"*
- *"Does it add any support to your new, alternative thought?"*
- *"Did you discover anything else?"*
- *"How could you apply this knowledge to improve things for you on a day-to-day basis?"*

Making future progress and overcoming problems

- *"Do you have any continuing doubts? How could you test these?"*
- *"How could you overcome any difficulties in future?"*
- *"What can you do next to continue to make progress?"*

Case Example 7.1: *Continued*: improving sleep patterns

Trisha concluded that she could cope without napping and that this did improve her night-time sleep, which made her less tired overall. She had also found that, by increasing activity instead of napping, she had managed to achieve more during her day, which gave her an increased sense of satisfaction.

Case Example 7.2: Overcoming procrastination

Keith is a journalist. He is often given a short deadline for completing articles. He became mildly depressed about 6 months ago and since then has had increasing difficulty meeting these deadlines. This has resulted in the following vicious cycles:

Thoughts:	I won't be able to write it properly.
	What if it's not good enough?
	I can't do this – I'm too anxious to even get started.
Feelings:	Anxious
	Low
Physical symptoms:	Tense, shaky
	Physically agitated – can't sit still
	Difficulty concentrating
Behaviour:	Puts off getting started until the last minute
	Eventually rushes through writing the article –
	standard may be lower

Keith's behavioural experiment planning chart

Thought being tested:	Just getting started by writing something about the subject, even if it is not very well written, might make me feel less anxious and help me write a better article
What am I going to do? (what, where, when…?)	For the next two weeks on alternate days, try the following two different strategies: 1. Continue current behaviour of putting off getting started until the last minute 2. Try a new strategy of doing 20 minutes of writing on the subject within an hour of receiving the brief; pay no attention to 'quality' of writing at this stage – just write something about the subject Every day I will monitor how quickly I finish writing the brief, how anxious I feel during the day and how well written I think the finished article is
What do I predict will happen?	I will spend 20 minutes writing complete rubbish and will feel even more frustrated afterwards
What problems might arise with this plan?	Anxiety or panic may overcome me and I might not get started as quickly as planned
How could these problems be overcome?	Turn computer on and sit at desk even if feeling anxious Try to ignore anxious thoughts/ feelings and just start writing anyway Avoid distractions (e.g. don't turn TV on)
What happened when I tried the experiment?	On the days that I was trying the new approach I sometimes found it difficult to sit down and get started with my work but once I actually started writing it became much easier. I finished the article more quickly and felt less anxious. The article was often better because I had more time to write it.
What have I learned from this experiment?	Just getting started with the article, by writing something about the subject, helps me to finish it more quickly, and it is sometimes of a higher standard than when I am rushed. It is better to write something down, even if it is not perfect.

Key learning points

- Changing unhelpful behaviour is one of the most important methods of breaking vicious cycles and making changes that have a genuine impact on daily life.
- It is often easier to 'do something differently' than to 'think differently'.
- Trying new behaviour can often provide evidence for alternative, balanced beliefs that makes them seem more credible.
- Encourage your patients to behave 'as if' they feel better or 'as if' they hold more balanced or helpful beliefs. This can set up a 'positive cycle' which reinforces and promotes positive change:

  "How would you behave if you felt more confident in this situation?"

  "What would you do if you were no longer depressed? What did you used to do differently?"

  "How do other people cope with this problem? Can you try that...?"

- Always break down behavioural changes into small, realistic and achievable steps which will build a patient's confidence and form building blocks for future change:

  "What might you do differently if you felt just a little better?"

- Watch out for 'yes, but...' responses to your suggestions. When you become aware of this, make an effort to *stop* making directive suggestions or giving advice. Instead, hand back responsibility to the patient.
- Remind your patients that they should expect to experience problems when carrying out behavioural experiments and to actively look for ways to overcome them:

  "How might you overcome this problem? What could you try here...?"

Chapter 8

Goal setting and overcoming resistance to change

Goal setting

Goal setting is a key skill in helping people to make important life changes which can be maintained in the long term. Goals are specific concrete steps towards a longer-term target or direction and should be 'SMART' (*Box 8.1*). For example, "*I will go for a 20 minute walk on Mondays, Wednesdays and Fridays after breakfast*" rather than "*I will do more exercise*".

Box 8.1

'SMART' criteria for goals

Specific: clear definition of what the patient is going to do

Measurable: easy to measure if the goal has been achieved or not

Achievable: practical and realistic that the patient will be able to carry it out

Relevant: useful and helpful to overcome the problem

Timely: has a clearly defined timescale for carrying out the task

---

Goals should be planned collaboratively with the patient. Don't set a patient's goals for them, because they are far less likely to follow the plan.

The next step is to plan how to achieve the goal. This involves deciding:

- **What?** — Make a phone call
- **Who with?** — My friend Maggie
- **Where?** — At home
- **How much / how long?** — Speak on the phone for 10 minutes
- **When?** — After breakfast
- **How often?** — Twice a week

Larger goals can be broken down into smaller steps or 'mini-goals' so that the patient can achieve something each week. For example, for a patient with a goal of increasing their exercise over the next two months:

Where I am now	STEP 1 Weeks 1–2	STEP 2 Weeks 3–4	STEP 3 Weeks 5–6	STEP 4 Weeks 7–8
I get a lift to the shop to buy my paper	Walk to the shop and get a lift back every day	Walk to the shop and get a lift back on two days this week	Walk to the shop and back taking 15 minutes each way	Walk to the shop and back taking 10 minutes each way

Encourage the patient to use a diary to record their goals. To avoid becoming overwhelmed, it is helpful to focus on one or two goals at a time. Try also to involve family and friends, who can offer praise and reinforce any changes made.

Values and personal benefits for making change

People will be more motivated if they can see a personal benefit for making a change. For example, you can ask:

"What are the benefits of increasing physical fitness for you?"

"How might being fitter make life better for you?"

Focusing on important life areas and values can also help individuals to identify what is really important to them and set their goals accordingly. In comparison to goals, which are specific and concrete, values are like directions on a compass. For example: being a good friend (value) versus phoning my friend once a week (goal).

Values are never 'achieved' but can influence the direction and clarify the purpose of an individual's life journey. They include principles, standards, qualities or activities that we consider worthwhile or important, and which bring meaning to our lives. Try asking:

"What is important to you in the big picture of your life?"

"What would you like your life to be about?"

"What goals can you set in the direction of these important areas?"

"How can stopping smoking help move you in your valued directions?"

It can be helpful first to identify the life areas that are important to a particular patient and then discuss their personal values and set specific goals accordingly (see *Box 8.2*).

Setting goals according to important life areas and values enables a flexible approach to making changes with the overall aim of improving an individual's life. Committing to action consistent with values recognises that there may be many possible solutions to a particular problem and thus encourages

Box 8.2

Examples of important life areas, values and possible goals

Life area	Examples of values	Examples of goals
Relationships with family and friends	Being a loving parent Caring for my spouse Being a good friend	Play football with my son at the weekend Take time to talk to my husband about his day Phone my friend each week
Work/school/education	To find a job that fits my skills and interests To be knowledgeable about the world To learn and develop new skills	Study for a new qualification Type up my CV Read the newspaper Start online French lessons
Hobbies/activities/helping others	To participate in a sport with others Being creative Helping others	Play football each Sunday Take a photography class Volunteer at the local charity shop
Emotional wellbeing and spirituality	Talking through problems and feelings with others Relaxation and 'me' time Religious and spiritual values	Talk to close friends about how I feel Have a long bath at the weekend Go to church at least every month
Caring for physical health	Keeping fit and active Eating a healthy diet Self-care of physical illnesses	Go swimming twice a week Eat healthy snacks instead of chocolate Take my medications as prescribed
Daily responsibilities	Taking care of my home and possessions Being organised Being dependable	Do the washing up Mend the broken fence in the garden Pay bills on time Use a diary to plan my week

brainstorming and problem-solving for different ways of moving in a valued direction.

Plan rewards

Planning rewards for achieving goals and any small successes can help motivate people to keep up the changes over time. A reward could be as simple as saying to yourself "*Well done!*", or it might involve a trip to the cinema or buying a favourite magazine. Rewards don't have to cost money; for example, taking time out for a relaxing bath or to read a book. Encourage patients to avoid unhealthy or counterproductive rewards, such as food high in fat and sugar.

> **Case Example 8.1: Planning rewards**
>
> Brian had recently given up smoking. He decided to save up the money that he would have spent on cigarettes each day. At the end of the month he was amazed by how much money he had saved and spent the money on some new CDs and DVDs.

Building confidence to achieve goals

It is very important to check that a patient feels confident that they will succeed with a particular goal. Ask:

"How confident are you that you can achieve this goal on a scale of 1–10?"

If a patient rates their confidence to change as five or less, then try to encourage them to set a more realistic or achievable goal.

You can also help to build a patient's confidence in their ability to make change by asking questions such as:

"What gives you confidence already? How could you build on this?"

"What achievements have you made in the past? What attitudes did you have? What actions did you take? How did you overcome any problems?"

"What would you do differently if you felt more confident? Can you start to behave 'as if' you felt a little more confident?"

"Can you get any inspiration or support from others?"

Overcoming barriers to change

There are many barriers and obstacles which can make it difficult to make or stick to changes (see *Box 8.3* for some common examples). It can be helpful to proactively discuss potential barriers with the patient in advance. Ask:

Box 8.3

Examples of barriers to making change

- Places and things, e.g. it may be harder to avoid daytime napping if you stay in the house and sit on the sofa
- People, e.g. spending time with smokers makes it difficult to quit smoking
- Thoughts and feelings, e.g. feeling depressed or demotivated makes it difficult to get out for a walk
- Physical symptoms, e.g. pain makes it difficult to be more active

"What might get in the way of achieving this goal?"

"How might you overcome that problem?"

Try turning the question around to help look for solutions. Ask the patient:

"What places or people make it easier for you to make this change?"

"What thoughts, attitudes or emotions make it easier to do this? How might you encourage these?"

You can also use problem-solving techniques (see *Chapter 9*) to help patients find solutions to overcome difficulties that arise with a particular goal.

Reviewing goals

Always review goals when you next see the patient. Make sure you congratulate and praise the patient for any progress, no matter how small, in order to reinforce and encourage continued change.

Goals should be regularly re-evaluated and increased over time. This should be a very slow and gradual process. Raising targets too quickly is likely to lead to setbacks and the patient may give up if it becomes too challenging too quickly.

Coping with setbacks

Successful change is rarely a smooth process and usually involves overcoming a variety of setbacks, and ups and downs. Encourage the patient not to get disheartened when they experience a setback, but to see it as an opportunity for learning (see *Box 8.4* for some strategies to cope with setbacks).

Strategies for overcoming setbacks

- Avoid 'risky' situations, for example, going to a pub when you are trying to cut down alcohol intake.
- Develop ways of coping when you are in a 'high-risk' situation, for example, plan a distraction activity such as phoning a friend when you feel the urge to have a cigarette.
- Don't give up completely when things go wrong. Remember that setbacks are inevitable. Simply drop back to an earlier stage and start again from there.
- Get some support – ask friends and family to help you keep up the changes. For added support you could also join a local group such as a weight loss or walking group.
- Remember to use a written diary to plan and record changes.
- Keep remembering to give yourself rewards and encouragement for making change.
- Remind yourself why the changes are important to you personally.

Pacing

The boom and bust cycle

Pacing is a strategy used to avoid a common problem known as 'boom and bust', which involves a vicious cycle of over- and under-activity (see *Figure 8.1*). Here, people tend to vary the amount of exercise or activity that they carry out according to how they feel, either physically or emotionally. This cycle is based on the unhelpful belief that it is necessary to rest or avoid activity completely when experiencing certain symptoms such as fatigue. Then on a 'good day' people carry out far more activity than planned in an attempt to

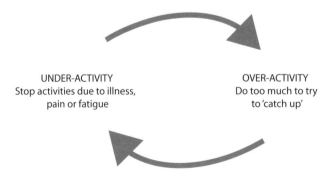

UNDER-ACTIVITY
Stop activities due to illness,
pain or fatigue

OVER-ACTIVITY
Do too much to try
to 'catch up'

Figure 8.1:   Boom and bust in relation to exercise

'catch up'. This leads to increased fatigue and risk of injury and leads to more rest in the following days to compensate. Overall, this pattern results in a general reduction in fitness and increased fatigue over time.

Case Example 8.2: Boom and bust

Joan had been trying to increase her activity levels in order to lose weight. She had been doing well for a few weeks but then came down with a cold. She felt frustrated because she wanted to buy her granddaughter a birthday present. Joan decided to rest for a week until over her cold, and as soon as she felt better, she went to the shopping centre and spent all day walking around the shops. Afterwards she felt exhausted with achy muscles. She needed to rest again for several days.

Pacing – an alternative to boom and bust

Rather than stopping activities altogether when feeling tired or unwell, pacing involves reducing activity to a planned baseline, from which the patient can gradually build back up when feeling better.

Case Example 8.2: *Continued*: an alternative pacing approach

Joan rested for the first two days of her cold and then restarted building up her exercise gradually in the garden and by walking to the local shop. Then, rather than trying to spend all day at the shopping centre, she took the bus to the local town centre for an hour and was able to find a present for her granddaughter. She felt well after this and was able to continue being active.

Motivational interviewing

Motivational interviewing (MI) is a very useful approach to supporting and encouraging patients to make changes such as losing weight, stopping smoking or reducing drug or alcohol consumption. MI has been shown to promote behaviour change and leads to better outcomes for patients in a variety of settings (Rubak *et al.*, 2005).

Making a life change is often difficult, and patients may seem ambivalent or lack motivation. Many health professionals react by offering prescriptive advice to make change using a directive communication style. Unfortunately, this often has the opposite effect and simply generates resistance ('yes, but...') or passivity in the patient, and makes it harder for them to change.

In MI, the health professional takes the stance of a well-informed guide. This involves engaging and working collaboratively with patients, emphasising their autonomy over decision-making, and eliciting their motivation for change. This approach fits well with the principles of communication that underlie CBT and the two methods work extremely well alongside one another.

Key communication skills for MI

This involves "Asking", "Listening" and "Informing" (Rollnick *et al.*, 2008):

- **"Ask"** open ended questions – invite the patient to consider how and why they might change.
- **"Listen"** and try to understand your patient's experience, using reflective and empathic statements that summarise their thoughts and beliefs. Don't lecture, argue or try to convince the patient to make a change. When faced by uncertainty or resistance, encourage the patient to reflect and discuss their views. This will lead to a better relationship and is more effective at promoting long-term change.
  "It sounds as if you would like to reduce your alcohol intake but you are finding it difficult to make the change..."
- **"Inform"** – ask permission to provide information, and then discuss what the implications might be for the patient.

Some additional useful strategies that can be used to guide and encourage behaviour change are described below.

Develop discrepancy

Motivation for change is encouraged by helping people to recognise that there is a gap or discrepancy between their current behaviour and their long-term goals or values (e.g. *I would like to be healthy for my grandchildren but I am continuing to smoke*). You can use reflective questions to help identify the discrepancy, such as:

"Tell me what concerns you about [your weight]?"

"Tell me what [smoking] has cost you?"

Discuss the importance of change

If a patient does not see a change as being important, they are unlikely to make much effort to carry it out. It is therefore important to establish whether this change is important to the individual patient. Ask questions such as:

"How important is it to you to [lose weight]...?"

"How might things be different if you...?"

"What are the biggest benefits if you make the change?"

A health professional may sometimes need to provide additional information about the importance of change. Make sure that you provide it in small manageable chunks and that you ask for feedback and check understanding after each step.

CHECK   *"What do you know about the benefits of stopping smoking...?"*

↓

CHUNK   *"Yes, you are right that smoking can cause lung cancer. There are many health benefits for stopping smoking. This can also reduce your risk of having a heart attack..."*

↓

CHECK   *"How do you think this might apply to you...?"*

Cost–benefit analysis

Discussing the pros and cons of changing or carrying out a cost-benefit analysis is also a useful method of encouraging change (see *Case Example 8.3*).

Case Example 8.3: Cost–benefit analysis of taking medication for hypertension

Mohammed is a 64 year old man with hypertension – his last blood pressure reading was 165/101. He is also a smoker. He has been prescribed anti-hypertensive medication but his blood pressure remains consistently high. During one surgery visit, he admits to his GP that he does not take his medication every day. His GP suggests that Mohammed makes a cost–benefit analysis of this behaviour:

Behaviour: missing doses of anti-hypertension medication

Advantages / benefits	Disadvantages / costs
"I don't like the unpleasant side-effects of taking the tablets" "Not taking it every day stops my body getting dependent on the medication" "I don't want my life to be ruled or controlled by having to take tablets every day"	"High blood pressure can increase my chances of getting seriously ill, like having a heart attack or a stroke" "It is important to me to remain as healthy as possible, for the sake of my wife and family" "Knowing my blood pressure is high makes me feel quite anxious" "I don't give my body a chance to get used to the medication – side-effects may settle down or I may get more used to them"

Advantages / benefits	Disadvantages / costs
	"I could switch medication if the side-effects are unbearable"
	"The doctor says that these tablets are not addictive"

Alternative perspective: taking my medication regularly might bring down my blood pressure and make me feel more in control of my health. It will also cut down my risk of getting seriously ill in the future.

How could I behave differently? Make an effort to take my medication every day, as prescribed. I will come and see the doctor if the tablets do not agree with me.

Notice and encourage 'change talk'

Pay close attention to when the patient uses language that suggests that they are considering change ('change talk'), such as:

> "I know I should stop smoking..."

> "I should try not to drink every day..."

When you notice change talk, try to highlight and reflect it back to the patient:

> "So you would like to stop smoking...? What makes it difficult for you...?"

> "Where does that leave you now?"

Emphasise autonomy

Always emphasise the patient's freedom of choice and highlight that the responsibility to make change lies with the patient. Remember, no matter how convincing you are, in the end it will always be the patient's own decision whether to change or not:

> "It is your decision as to when and how you might make any change"

> "How might you see yourself getting started with this...?"

Case Example 8.4: Overcoming resistance to change

Donald is a 56 year old diabetic who has come to see his GP. His diabetes control is very poor and he is overweight. He has recently been made redundant and finds it difficult to motivate himself to get anything done. He says he has only come to stop his wife 'nagging'.

GP	OK, let's talk though the issues that you are facing. You probably know that losing some weight and getting more exercise will help your diabetes and your health, but what do you feel about this?
Donald	I don't know doctor. It's all a bit much really.
GP	It sounds like you are feeling a bit overwhelmed by this?
Donald	Well, it's not easy you know. I'm fed up with this diabetes.
GP	It sounds like it's getting you down a bit. I'm sorry to hear that.
Donald	Every time I come to the doctor I get told I have to do something different.
GP	That must be difficult. I wonder if there is any part of you that would like to make any of these changes?
Donald	Well, I'd like to get my sugars better and of course I'd like to lose weight. But it's not easy.
GP	No, I can understand that. Can you tell me why you think it might be important for you to lose some weight?
Donald	I know it's not good for my diabetes. And my knees are aching. I think it might be arthritis.
GP	Yes, that's all very true. Losing weight has a lot of health benefits, including improving your sugars and the risk of arthritis in your knees.
Donald	Well yes, but nothing I do seems to help.
GP	So, you are trying to lose weight but finding it a challenge?
Donald	I'm not sure I'll ever get there.
GP	You sound a little demoralised.
Donald	I suppose I am. I really do want to lose weight but I do a job where I sit down all day and it's hard to find the time for exercise.
GP	So you do want to lose weight but it's hard to find the time to exercise when you do a sedentary job?
Donald	Yes.
GP	Have you had any thoughts as to how you might increase your activity levels?
Donald	I'm not sure, I hate the gym!
GP	So not the gym! Have you ever been more active in the past?
Donald	I used to do a bit of walking at weekends when I had more time.

GP   Walking has been shown to be a very beneficial exercise for
          strengthening the heart and for weight loss. Would you consider trying
          to build that up once more?

Donald   I suppose so, although I don't know if I've got the time.

GP   It sounds like time pressure is a big issue for you. It's essential that
          any changes fit with your lifestyle and commitments. I wonder how
          important it might be to find some time for this?

Donald   Well, you are right. It is important. I suppose I could try to walk a bit
          more.

GP   That sounds like a great idea! Would you be willing to try to set some
          goals for increasing your walking...?

Key learning points

- Goal setting is a key skill for encouraging patients to make important life changes. Remember goals should be specific (who, what, when, where) and easily achievable.
- Don't forget to ask the patient how they got on with their goal when you next see them. It helps to write down what they plan to do – you can keep one copy and give another to the patient.
- Identifying the personal benefits of making a change can help motivate individuals. Take time to explore each patient's personal values and important life areas before planning relevant goals.
- Obstacles and setbacks are inevitable when making life changes, so encourage the patient to plan how they will cope with any potential difficulties, and discuss how to use pacing to avoid the boom–bust cycle.
- If the patient seems resistant to making changes, resist the temptation to try to convince them to change, or offer more suggestions or prescriptive advice, because this usually has the reverse effect of making an individual more entrenched in their beliefs and less likely to change.
- If you become aware of resistance then try some alternative approaches to encouraging change:
  - 'Roll with resistance' – don't confront but instead ask open questions to explore the patient's beliefs and ideas about making change. Reflect back what they say non-judgementally using empathic statements to build rapport.
  - Ask how important it is for the patient to make the change.

- ○ Highlight any conflict between their current behaviour and their long-term goals or values. Use a handover question to ask the patient to reflect on this.
- ○ Use a cost–benefit analysis to explore the pros and cons of making a change.
- ○ Emphasise patient autonomy and freedom of choice to change (or not).

Chapter 9

Overcoming practical problems: problem-solving approaches

What is 'problem-solving'?

Problem-solving techniques offer a structured way to overcome practical problems and make changes in challenging environmental circumstances.

The benefit of problem-solving approaches does *not* depend entirely on solving the patient's problems. It can be therapeutic simply to identify what the problems actually are, making life seem more understandable and manageable. Using a problem-solving approach can give people a sense of hope, as well as an increased sense of control over their lives and problems.

When to use a problem-solving approach

A problem-solving approach is useful when patients attribute many of their difficulties to the presence of practical problems and life stresses. Having to face a number of seemingly impossible problems can result in feelings of depression or anxiety.

A problem-solving approach can be combined with other strategies, such as altering unhelpful thoughts or behaviours that may be contributing to problems.

Introducing problem-solving to patients

Try to give a clear rationale and explanation of the problem-solving approach, because patients may already have unsuccessfully attempted to solve problems themselves or view them as completely impossible to change. This includes a brief overview of the approach and how it may help the patient:

> "Sometimes the problems in our lives can make us feel down or low, and make life seem overwhelming or out of control. This approach can help to make sense of these problems and look for solutions to them. Problem-solving might help you feel more in control of your life and lift your mood."

It is helpful to take a structured approach to problem-solving, which involves eight steps (*Box 9.1*).

Box 9.1

The eight steps of problem-solving

1. Make a list of problems.
2. Choose a problem to work on.
3. Define the problem clearly.
4. Generate solutions to the problem.
5. Choose a solution.
6. Make an action plan.
7. Carry out the plan.
8. Review what happened.

Patients should take an active role in the process and generate their own potential solutions to problems.

> *"As these are your problems, you understand them better than anyone else. You are the most important person in this process, and it is vital that you do the 'work' by finding your own ideas and suggestions."*

The Eight Steps of Problem-Solving

Step 1: Make a list of problems

The first step involves identifying and making a written list of the patient's different problems.

> *"What problems are bothering you the most at the moment?"*

The aim is to get a broad overview of the important areas without going into too much detail.

> *"OK, you mentioned that you have some financial troubles and also that you are not getting on too well with your husband. Are there any other important problems in your life at the moment?"*

The list should cover most key problem areas. It should include minor as well as major difficulties, because it may be helpful to focus on solving easier problems first.

It is often useful to discover how these problems are affecting the patient. This helps to provide motivation to make changes. Remember to express empathy for the emotional distress associated with a patient's difficult life problems.

> *"How are these problems affecting your life? How do they make you feel?"*

> *"That sounds really difficult. It must be very distressing for you."*

Once the problem list is complete, give the patient a brief summary of what they have told you.

> *"We have made a list of the practical problems that you are facing at the moment. You are having financial troubles with your mortgage, problems in your relationship with your partner, and you have a difficult boss at work."*

> *"Tell me, have I got this right...?"*

Case Example 9.1: Making a list of problems

Karen is a 27 year old nurse, who works part-time on a surgical ward in the local hospital. She has become depressed over the past year. She is married and has two children aged 2 and 5. Karen's GP suggests trying a problem-solving approach to understand and resolve some of the difficulties that she faces. They begin by generating Karen's current problem list:

1. Unhappy at work – doesn't get on with ward manager.
2. No time for herself – lack of enjoyable activities in her life.
3. Health problems – recurrent back pain.
4. Husband facing possible redundancy which would cause the family major financial difficulties.

Step 2: Choose a problem to solve

The next step is for the patient to choose a problem to focus on first.

> *"Which of these problems would you be most interested in looking at in more depth?"*

For problem-solving to be effective, the problem must:
- involve an area which it is possible for the patient to change
- be important to the patient.

It is not necessary to choose the most complex or difficult problem on the list.

> *"For the first attempt, it may be more helpful to choose a problem that is not too difficult, so that we are likely to be able to make some progress with it. This helps you to learn the technique and builds your confidence in using the approach."*

Successful problem-solving generally involves focusing on one problem at a time. However, some patients may feel that this it is not 'enough'. You could use guided discovery to discuss this issue and enable the patient to come to their own conclusions.

Case Example 9.1: *Continued*: choosing a problem to solve

Let's return to the example of Karen, the nurse with mild depression. In the following dialogue, Karen and her GP discuss the pros and cons of changing one problem at a time:

GP	Would you like to choose one of these problems to try to solve first?
Karen	I'm not sure. I have so many problems, I'm not sure that changing one small thing will make any difference.
GP	It sounds like you are thinking that *'Changing one small thing won't make any difference to my problems.'*
Karen	Yes, that's right.
GP	What makes you think that is true?
Karen	I have so many problems at the moment. There doesn't seem much point in just looking at one small area.
GP	OK – I will write that down. Anything else that makes you think that way?
Karen	I feel so fed up, I'm not sure I can change anything anyway.
GP	That's important to know. Any more reasons why *'changing one thing won't make any difference'?*
Karen	Well… some of the most important problems might not be possible to solve – I can't give my husband a new job, for example.
GP	I understand. I have written all these reasons down. Now, can you think of anything that might challenge or contradict the idea that *'changing one thing won't make any difference'?* Is it possible that it could help in any way?
Karen	I suppose that it is still better to solve some problems, even if I can't solve them all.
GP	Excellent. Anything else?
Karen	I'm not sure.
GP	How might it make you feel, to successfully solve some of your problems, even small ones?
Karen	I would probably feel quite pleased with myself.
GP	Yes, hopefully it would build up your confidence and boost your mood a bit. Do you think there might be any advantage in looking at one problem at a time? What might be the difficulties in trying to solve all your problems at once?
Karen	It is probably impossible to solve everything at once. I probably wouldn't get very far and I might just give up and feel worse.
GP	Great. Could you read through the evidence you have thought up, for

> | | and against the idea that 'changing one thing won't make any difference to my problems'. What do you make of all this now? |
> |---|---|
> | Karen | I can see that it does make sense to try to work on one thing at a time and that even improving one small thing might boost my spirits. |
> | GP | Yes, that makes a lot of sense. Now, which problem would you like to look at first? Ideally, it should be something important to you and possible to change… |
> | Karen | I am not very happy at work. Perhaps we should look at that. |
> | GP | OK, let's move onto the next step and talk about it in more depth… |

Step 3: Define the problem clearly

The problem must be clearly defined in precise and simple terms. It should be focused, specific and not too complex. Patients will often initially describe very broad, general problem areas. However, it is often helpful to break these down into smaller, more manageable chunks:

General / broad problem: I am lonely and depressed

⬇   ⬇

Specific / focused / clear: I don't go out to any social events during the week

Encourage the patient to identify what specific 'chunks' would be most useful to look at first.

> *"You have described your problem in quite general terms. It is often easier to solve a problem by breaking it down into smaller 'chunks' and working through one at a time."*

For example, a patient may describe a problem of 'not having a girlfriend'. It might be helpful to break this down into specific areas, such as:
- Lack of social interaction (e.g. few friends or lack of regular social activities).
- Not meeting single women because of current lifestyle (e.g. working long hours).
- Lack of self-confidence (e.g. avoids talking to members of the opposite sex, anxiety about personal attributes or attractiveness).

Case Example 9.1: *Continued*: **defining problems clearly**

Let's return again to the example of Karen. In the following dialogue, Karen and her GP discuss her work problems in order to define the problem clearly.

GP	You mentioned your problems with work. Could you be a bit more specific about what exactly you find difficult?
Karen	The main problem is that I don't have a good relationship with my ward manager. We are very short-staffed and she expects us to do extra shifts without much notice. But I can't do that because I can't get childcare.
GP	Is there anything else?
Karen	Well, the manager can be quite bossy and critical. Several of my good friends have left the nursing team in the past year so I am not really enjoying working on that ward any more.
GP	I see. I made a note of the areas that you mentioned: you have a difficult relationship with your ward manager, the ward is short-staffed, you are expected to do extra shifts without notice, you find your manager bossy and critical, and several of your friends have left the team in the past year. Is that right?
Karen	Yes, that's it.
GP	What would you like to achieve from solving this problem? What specific areas would you like to improve?
Karen	I would like to enjoy my work again and have good relationships with my colleagues.
GP	Great. I will make a note of that.

Step 4: Generate solutions to problems

The next stage is to encourage the patient to think of a wide range of potential solutions to their problem. The patient must take an active role in leading the discussion and generating solutions. First the patient must consider **what** they would like to achieve:

"What would need to change for you to feel better...?"

Next, the patient must think creatively, or 'brainstorm' possible solutions for **how** to achieve this goal. The more solutions that are generated, the more likely a useful one will emerge. It is therefore useful to include a wide range of potential solutions, even if some ideas seem impractical or ridiculous. These 'wild' solutions could be adapted or modified to become workable, realistic possibilities.

"Can you think of any possible solutions to this problem?"

"What other ideas can you think of? Try to think of as many possibilities as you can..."

"What would your best friend/partner/boss/parent suggest? What advice would you give to a friend in the same situation?"

"Can you think of any ridiculous or 'crazy' solutions as well as more sensible ones?"

From *theory* to *practice*...	Encourage lateral thinking using the 'brick technique' (Nezu & Nezu, 1989) to help patients to think creatively and laterally about new ways to solve problems.
	Ask the patient to think up as many uses as possible for an item such as a house brick.
	Initially, the patient is likely to generate common, obvious suggestions such as building a house or a wall.
	Next, give the patient some other scenarios, to encourage them to think more laterally:
	• *"Could it have any other, more unusual uses?"* • *"Could it be used as a piece of furniture?"* • *"How would it be useful if you were trying to escape an attacker?"* • *"What if you became locked out of your car?"* • *"How might a child play with it?"*

Case Example 9.1: *Continued*: generating solutions to problems

Let's return to the example of Karen again. Her GP encourages Karen to 'brainstorm' a wide range of possible solutions to her problem with work.

GP	Can you think of any possible solutions to this problem?
Karen	I'm not sure. I suppose I could try to work shifts where the ward manager is not on duty.
GP	That's a good start. Anything else?
Karen	I could look for a job on a different ward.
GP	Good. What advice would you give to someone else in the same situation?
Karen	I might suggest that they discuss their childcare difficulties with their manager.

GP	OK, can you think of any really crazy or wild solutions to the problem? How else could you make your work more enjoyable?
Karen	Err… Well, I used to really enjoy chatting and laughing with my friends at work. I could throw a big party for all the ward staff to cheer them up!
GP	Great! Now, does that lead you to any other solutions which might help?
Karen	Actually, it might help me to get to know some of the new staff on the ward a bit better, maybe some kind of ward social event. We used to have them all the time.
GP	What exactly could you do to make this happen?
Karen	I could organise a ward night out. Or perhaps just invite a couple of the girls out for a drink after one of our shifts.

Step 5: Choose a solution

Once the patient has written a list of potential solutions, the next step is to consider each solution's advantages and disadvantages, in order to decide what action to take.

Box 9.2

Assessing the value of potential solutions

- How realistic or achievable is this solution likely to be?
- How helpful is this solution likely to be?
- What are the pros and cons of each suggestion (e.g. time, effort, money, stress or other emotional distress)?
- What positive or negative impact might this solution have on friends or family?

Again, most of these ideas should be generated by the patient. However, if the patient is overlooking a major advantage or disadvantage, then it can be helpful to bring it to their attention:

"Do you think it is important to take into account that....?"

After assessing each solution in turn, the patient must then choose the preferred solution(s) to try. Remember to check that the solutions are 'SMART' (see *Chapter 8*) because this helps to ensure that the solution is realistic, workable and potentially useful for solving the patient's problem.

If the patient's chosen solutions seem overambitious, it may be helpful to encourage them to break them down into smaller, more achievable 'chunks':

> "This is a very interesting solution, but I am concerned it may be quite difficult for you to achieve it all at once. Can you see any way to break it down into smaller pieces that might be easier to manage?"

Overly complex solutions may also indicate that the problem definition itself is too broad. In this case, return to *Step 3* and break down the problem further into smaller sections or stages, which can be approached individually.

Case Example 9.1: *Continued*: assessing the advantages and disadvantages of solutions

Returning again to Karen, here is a list of her solutions.

Solution	Advantages	Disadvantages
Try to work shifts when ward manager is not on duty	Avoid being criticised or asked to work extra shifts	Difficult to manage – manager organises rota
Look for another job on a different ward	New challenges Potentially better work environment	May be worse than current job Have to get to know new environment / system Might be stressful
Discuss childcare issues with ward manager	May stop her making unrealistic demands on my time Quick	Scary to talk to her – she could get angry Might not make any difference
Throw a big party for ward staff	Fun	Expensive Too much organisation
Organise a ward night out	Get to know ward staff better	What if no one came? Difficult to coordinate with shifts of all staff
Invite a few people for a drink after work	Nice to get to know people Might make work more enjoyable if make friends	They might not want to come Would I be able to arrange childcare?

Choice of solution(s):

1. Discuss childcare issues with ward manager.
2. Invite two people (Amanda and Jane) for coffee after work.

Step 6: Make an action plan

Once the solution has been chosen, the next stage is to draw up a written action plan and, being as specific as possible, write down exactly *what* the patient plans to do and *when* (*Box 9.3*).

Box 9.3

Steps for making an action plan

- What needs to be done?
- Where is it to be done?
- Who does it involve?
- How will it be done?
- When will it be done?
- What difficulties might arise and how will I cope with them?

Patients must understand what they need to do and feel comfortable and confident enough to try the solution out in practice.

"Are you clear about what you are going to do?"

"How confident are you that you will be able to carry this out?"

If they lack confidence in achieving the plan, the solution may need to be broken down into simpler steps.

"How could we change this plan to make it seem more manageable or realistic for you to achieve?"

It can also be helpful to consider what barriers might prevent patients from achieving a particular plan and to plan in advance how to overcome them.

"What might get in the way of being able to achieve this?"

"How could you overcome these difficulties?"

As with any other 'homework' task, it is important to establish a patient's commitment to carrying out the plan. Health professionals can encourage patients by expressing interest in the outcome of the task, both beforehand and in a review consultation afterwards.

"Carrying out the plan is the most important step, because it can improve your problems. I will be really interested in hearing how you got on when I see you again in two weeks."

It is helpful to create a *written* action plan, with a copy for both GP and patient to keep.

Case Example 9.1: *Continued*: turning solutions into plans

Following on from before, here is Karen's action plan.

Solution	Action plan
Discuss childcare issues with ward manager	*Plan* • Ring ward manager in advance and ask her to arrange a time to discuss rota • Explain difficulties with childcare and not able to do many 'ad hoc' shifts – request rota in advance to book childcare arrangements *Possible difficulties* • Might feel nervous and get tongue-tied *How to overcome difficulties* • Plan what to say in advance and write it down
Invite two people (Amanda and Jane) for coffee	*Plan* • Look for a shift when both Amanda and Jane are on duty within the next week or so • Suggest going for coffee after one morning shift in the next 2–3 weeks *Possible difficulties* • They might be busy or say no • Might not fit with my childcare arrangements *How to overcome difficulties* • Be flexible about date, time and location • Be prepared to have coffee with one of them instead of both on the first occasion (could repeat another time if it goes well)

Step 7: Carry out the plan

This is a self-explanatory step where the patient carries out the action plan.

Step 8: Review what happened

One of the most important stages of problem-solving is to reflect on what actually happened after trying out a solution. Always remember to ask patients how they got on with any agreed solution or action plan (*Box 9.4*). This gives a clear message that trying out the plan is important and necessary to solve problems.

"What happened when you tried…? I am really interested to hear about it."

Box 9.4

Questions for reviewing the outcome of problem-solving action plans

- What did the patient do?
- Did it help to improve the problem? How?
- Were there any other positive outcomes?
- Were there any problems or difficulties with the approach?
- What can the patient learn from this?

To boost a patient's confidence and belief in their ability to make change, remember to emphasise and praise *any* success or positive outcome, however small.

Reviewing difficulties

If the patient found the action plan difficult to carry out or unhelpful in solving their problem, it is important to review these difficulties (*Box 9.5*). Any difficulties encountered should be viewed as 'learning opportunities' rather than as 'failures'.

Box 9.5

Reviewing difficulties with problem-solving

1. **If the action plan was too difficult or the patient was unable to carry it out, ask:**
- Was the plan too ambitious or unrealistic?
- What obstacles got in the way? How could these be overcome?
- Did the patient lack motivation for the task? How could this be increased in future? What benefits might arise from solving this problem?
- Was the problem less important than other issues in the patient's life that should be addressed first?

2. **If the plan was not helpful for solving the problem, consider:**
- Was the patient attempting to change something that was outside their control?
- Was the solution not focused on the most important part of the problem for the patient?
- Is the problem still important to solve? If so, how could the patient change their approach to the problem?

Case Example 9.1: *Continued*: reviewing what happened

Karen returns to see her GP two weeks after trying out the problem-solving approach, to discuss what happened.

GP	I am very interested to find out what happened with your plan to try to solve your problems at work…
Karen	Well, I did try to carry out the plan that we agreed, but it wasn't very easy. I put it off until I knew I was coming back to see you!
GP	It can sometimes be difficult to make changes. What happened?
Karen	I was planning to do two things. One of them was quite easy. About 3 days after I saw you, I noticed that Jane and Amanda were both on duty with me. During our break, I suggested that we went for a coffee one day after work.
GP	How did they respond to that?
Karen	They both said they would really like to. They seemed pleased and we are due to go to a café next Wednesday. My husband has agreed to look after my children for a couple of hours, so it should be no problem.
GP	Great. How do you feel about this? Has it helped solve your problem with work at all?
Karen	I'm pleased because I made the effort and it worked out. I hope that it might make work a bit more enjoyable if I know these people better.
GP	Was it helpful in any other way at all?
Karen	It will be nice to get my social life a bit more active, now that some of my friends have moved away from the area.
GP	I am pleased that went well. What does this show you about your ability to solve your problems and improve life?
Karen	It shows that I can make a difference, as long as I actually make the effort to do things.
GP	I think that's absolutely right. You mentioned that the other part of the plan wasn't so easy. What happened?
Karen	I was supposed to talk to my ward manager about my childcare problems but I didn't get around to it.
GP	What stopped you from doing this?
Karen	Well, she was away on holiday for the first week. Then, I didn't see her at all for quite a few days. By then, I had lost my nerve!
GP	What do you mean by 'losing your nerve'? What were you concerned might happen?
Karen	I was worried that she would get angry and shout at me.
GP	I see. Is it still important to you to have this discussion with her?

Karen	It is important because I want to make it clear that I just can't do all these extra shifts. I'm getting really stressed every time I see the rota and I want to sort it out.
GP	So it is still something important to you to change?
Karen	Yes it is.
GP	How could you overcome this problem with 'losing your nerve'? What might help?
Karen	I think it might help if I don't keep putting it off. She is back from holiday now so I should phone up and arrange to see her very soon.
GP	Anything else?
Karen	I could practise what I am going to say and write it down. I didn't do that last time.
GP	Great. Is there any way to look at the situation that might make it seem less intimidating or scary?
Karen	Well, I could imagine her naked!
GP	That might work! How likely do you think it is that she will shout at you?
Karen	Well, she might not shout at me at all.
GP	Would it still be worth doing, even if she did get angry and shout at you?
Karen	Yes I think so, because this is a problem that is important to sort out. If she really is that unreasonable I would have to think more seriously about changing to a different ward.
GP	I see. Let's make another action plan…

The problem-solving cycle

Problem-solving can be seen as an ongoing cycle of identifying problems, looking for solutions, and then reviewing the outcome of any changes made (*Figure 9.1*).

The approach helps to encourage individual resilience in the face of difficulties, by recognising that there may never be an 'absolute' solution to problems, but that life involves a continuous process of reflecting on difficulties and looking for solutions.

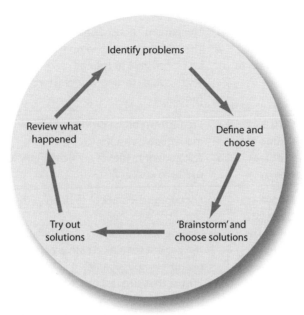

Figure 9.1:   The problem-solving cycle

Key learning points

- Problem-solving techniques offer a structured way to understand and overcome practical or environmental problems.
- It is not necessary to solve all the problems for a patient to feel better – the process of identifying and clarifying problems can be therapeutic in itself, by making difficulties seem more manageable and increasing their sense of control over life.
- The approach promotes an attitude of resilience where individuals are able to identify and reflect on difficulties and seek ways to overcome them.
- Always encourage a patient to take responsibility for solving their own problems.

Summary of the stages of problem-solving

Step 1 – Make a list of problems	<ul><li>Make a written list of all important problems</li><li>Include more simple / minor problems as well as complex / major problems</li></ul>
	<ul><li>Ask how the problems are affecting a patient's life; this can help build motivation to make potentially difficult changes</li><li>Express empathy for difficulties and emotional distress</li><li>Finish with a brief summary of the problem list</li></ul>

Step 2 – Choose a problem to solve	• The patient chooses one problem area to focus on • The problem must be important to the patient as well as being possible to change • Try to avoid starting with the most complex or difficult problems
Step 3 – Define the problem clearly	• Break down broad problem areas into smaller, more manageable chunks • Ask patient to identify which 'chunk' it would be most useful to look at first
Step 4 – Generate solutions to the problem	• Encourage the patient to brainstorm a wide range of potential solutions • Include some impractical or ridiculous ideas as this helps the patient to think creatively and may lead to some useful, new possibilities • Ensure that suggestions are being generated by the patient
Step 5 – Choose a solution	• Ask patients to identify the advantages and disadvantages of each potential solution to the problem • Next, patients should choose their preferred solution(s) to try • Check that solutions fit the 'SMART' criteria and are realistic, achievable and useful
Step 6 – Make an action plan	• Draw up a clear written action plan of what they are planning to try • Discuss in advance what difficulties might arise with the plan and how to overcome them • Offering a follow-up appointment may help motivate the patient to carry out the task
Step 7 – Carry out the plan	
Step 8 – Review what happened	• Review what happened after trying out a solution to a problem • Reinforce and encourage *any* positive success to help motivate patients to persist when making changes • Reflect on any difficulties that arose and try to identify ways to overcome these barriers to solving the problem • Plan the next steps

Chapter 10

Deeper levels of belief: core beliefs and rules

Different types of thought

CBT identifies three different levels of thought process: automatic thoughts, 'rules for living' and 'core beliefs' (*Figure 10.1*).

Automatic thoughts are the most 'superficial' level of thought. These are the most accessible and easily identifiable type of thoughts, which 'pop' into people's minds throughout the day.

In disorders such as depression, negative automatic thoughts can be compared to the growth of weeds in a garden (Greenberger & Padesky, 1995b). Learning to evaluate and find rational alternatives for negative thoughts is like cutting down these weeds, allowing the flowers (helpful, alternative thoughts) to grow through. For many patients, this process is enough to learn to cope with their problems effectively.

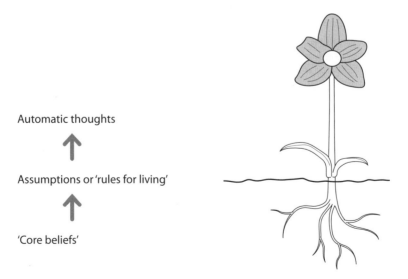

Automatic thoughts

↑

Assumptions or 'rules for living'

↑

'Core beliefs'

Figure 10.1: Different types of thought

However, negative automatic thoughts may reflect underlying, deeper levels of belief that people hold about themselves, other people and the world. It is sometimes necessary to remove weeds more permanently by digging down and taking them out by the root.

The deepest level thoughts are known as 'core beliefs'. These include both positive and negative views of the self and the world. Core beliefs typically involve absolutist statements that are expressed in black and white language such as:

I'm stupid	*I'm clever*
I'm worthless	*I'm interesting*
I'm weak and vulnerable to illness	*I'm strong and healthy*
Others are not to be trusted	*Others are kind and supportive*
The world is a dangerous place	*Things always turn out well*

'Rules for living' are a set of rules that guide people's expectations of themselves and others. They can often be expressed as 'should' statements or as conditional, 'if... then...' statements.

I should never make any mistakes

If I feel any physical symptoms then it means there is something seriously wrong

If I don't please others at all times then they will reject me

If people don't agree with me then it means that they don't respect me

I should always be in control

'Rules for living' often develop in order to help people live with 'tyrannical', absolutist, negative core beliefs. There are often two paired beliefs for each rule, which illustrate a person's beliefs about how they 'should' behave, as well as outlining the consequences or meaning if the rule is broken. For example, a person with the negative core belief *'I'm a failure'* may develop the following pair of rules:

If I do everything perfectly then it means that I am OK

If I make a mistake it means I am a total failure

Whilst automatic thoughts are often stated directly in people's minds, rules for living may be less obvious. However, they can often be inferred from people's actions or reactions to particular situations. People are often not consciously aware of the rules themselves, but are aware of the emotional discomfort that arises from transgressing them. If people's rules are, or are *at risk* of, being broken, they are likely to develop a negative emotional response associated with a host of negative automatic thoughts. This explains an apparent 'over-reaction' that a person may experience when faced by a seemingly minor event. For example, if someone holds perfectionist beliefs about potential failure, they are likely to feel extremely anxious in situations where this rule is threatened, such as taking an exam or any situation where they perceive there is a possibility of making a mistake. They may react by *avoiding* such situations or alternatively by working excessively hard to try to ensure continual 'success'.

Case Example 10.1: The development of core beliefs and rules for living

Anna was a quiet child. She was slightly overweight and wore glasses. She was often teased by the other children at school, who called her 'Specky-four-eyes'. Anna worked hard at school and often achieved good grades. However, whenever she was praised by teachers, her classmates would tease her, saying she was a 'boring, stuck-up, teacher's pet'.

Anna developed the core belief: *I am unacceptable to others.*

As she became older, Anna remained shy but developed a number of friendships. In response to these new experiences, she developed the following 'rules for living':

If someone doesn't like me then it means that I'm unacceptable

If everyone likes me then it means that I am OK

These rules make it easier for Anna to cope with her negative core belief. So long as (she perceives that) everyone likes her then she is able to believe that her core belief is not true. However, if this rule is threatened or broken then she returns to believing her negative, 'bottom line' belief of being unacceptable.

Because of her beliefs, Anna is vulnerable to feeling especially low or upset whenever she suspects that someone might not like her. To prevent this, she avoids threatening situations, such as meeting new people. She feels anxious and uncomfortable in social situations and experiences many negative, automatic thoughts about her own performance and the reactions of others such as:

Did I say something stupid?

I don't have anything interesting to say to anyone

This person thinks I am too quiet and boring

I should just go home – there is no point being here

In the early stages of CBT, Anna found that she continued to feel anxious in social situations, despite working on these automatic thoughts. It was therefore helpful to move on to learning some methods of gradually changing the rules and core beliefs that underlie her difficulties.

Where do rules and core beliefs come from?

Rules and core beliefs usually arise from early or past experiences. Children learn to make sense of their world by categorising their experiences into familiar patterns using language. The particular environment in which a child develops plays a strong role in shaping which beliefs are developed. For example, depending on their early experiences, a child may acquire beliefs such as either *dogs will bite* or *dogs are friendly.*

The simplistic, absolutist quality of core beliefs reflects this kind of early, childhood learning. Although these beliefs are not necessarily *absolutely* true, young children tend to view them as absolute fact. Children may also view subjective statements about themselves or others (e.g. *I am bad*), as being just as certain or 'true' as other, more factually based beliefs (e.g. *fire is dangerous*).

In later life, we learn to view most of these beliefs more flexibly. For example, we learn to approach dogs that are wagging their tails and avoid those that are growling. However, some of the old, absolute beliefs may remain. This is particularly likely if they developed from particularly traumatic experiences or if the beliefs are reinforced by ongoing life events.

Understanding how particular core beliefs and rules operate in individual patients can help to predict reactions or explain recurring themes of emotional distress in response to particular types of situation. The development of these beliefs is illustrated in *Figure 10.2.*

Unhelpful rules and core beliefs

Rules and core beliefs help people to generalise from experiences and make sense of new situations. For example, after learning to drive, we are able to drive a new, unfamiliar car with little difficulty. However, if we get in a car which is markedly *different,* such as one which is left-hand drive, we may make mistakes because our *old* knowledge of driving is not fully applicable within the new environment. The more ingrained the knowledge, the more difficult it is to adjust to new circumstances.

Core beliefs and rules are often *functional* and *adaptive* when they first develop. For example, a child who grows up in a violent, abusive or unpredictable environment may believe that *bad things that happen are my fault* and *if I don't do anything wrong then bad things may not happen.* These beliefs may help the child to cope in that environment, rather than risking further abuse or rejection from his parents. Blaming themselves for negative events around them may also give children a sense of control which may be preferable to feeling helpless and powerless. There may be an increased sense of security for children in believing that adults are 'good', even if this entails viewing themselves as 'bad'.

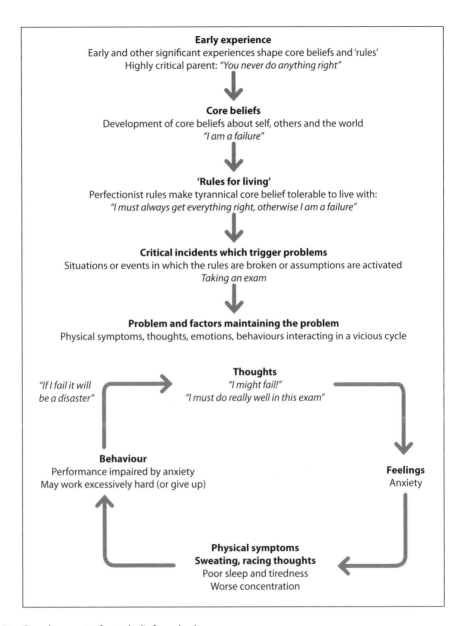

Figure 10.2: Development of core beliefs and rules

Core beliefs and rules are viewed as *dysfunctional* or *unhelpful* if they exert a negative or unhelpful effect on the person's life. On the whole, the more extreme and autocratic the rule, the less helpful it is likely to be. Dysfunctional beliefs arise when beliefs or rules are not adjusted or revised in the face of new evidence from later experience. Early beliefs may persist despite no longer being fully applicable to people's ongoing environment and circumstances. Such beliefs should be viewed as 'out of date' or 'unhelpful' rather than 'wrong'.

For many people, negative core beliefs and rules are activated only at certain times, such as periods of stress, low mood or in the presence of strong psychosocial pressures. However, in some enduring disorders, such as personality disorders, powerful, negative core beliefs and rules are typically active most of the time.

'Self-fulfilment' of rules and core beliefs

Holding a particular rule or core belief is usually 'self-fulfilling' because people behave '*as if*' the belief is absolute fact. For example, a woman who holds the rule, *I must always put others ahead of me so they don't see what a bad person I am,* is likely to behave in ways that that allow other people to dominate her or treat her as a 'doormat'. This serves to reinforce her belief that others think she is a bad person.

This also prevents people from testing out the possibility that the negative belief may not actually be true. For example, the belief that *if I spend time with others they will discover how boring I am and reject me,* may lead to avoidance of contact or interaction with other people. This means that the person is never able to discover that the rule is not entirely accurate.

Core beliefs and rules usually have an absolute, black and white content, which rarely fits the reality of the world. It is almost impossible to be a *total* failure or *completely* worthless. The beliefs are maintained by distorting the facts to fit the belief and by ignoring contradictory information. For example, a belief that *I am inferior to others* is usually based on numerous examples from someone's life, such as times that they have been ignored or badly treated by others. Someone holding this type of belief is likely to be highly sensitive and quick to notice experiences that confirm this perceived inferiority. They also tend to discount or ignore numerous examples of contradictory information.

Similarly, a perfectionist may achieve 99% in an exam but still agonise about the perceived 'failure' of that additional 1%. Padesky (1993) viewed this type of belief as an example of *self-prejudice.*

Case Example 10.2: Viewing unhelpful beliefs as 'self-prejudice'

In the following dialogue, Valerie and her GP discuss her negative self-beliefs.

GP   You mentioned that you are sometimes very critical of yourself, much more so than with other people. If even small things go wrong, you often view yourself as a 'complete failure'.

Valerie   Yes, that's right. I am very hard on myself.

GP   One way to look at this is to see it as a form of 'prejudice'. Imagine for a moment, a very sexist man who believes that *all* women drivers are

	terrible. One day he is walking down the street and he sees a woman driver having difficulty parking her car. She finishes by crashing into the car ahead. What would be his likely reaction?
Valerie	He would probably say, *"That's typical of a woman driver. They can't park. They shouldn't be on the road!"*
GP	Yes, that's right. It would confirm his idea that all women are bad drivers. The next day, this same man is walking down the road, when a woman does a perfect reverse park into a space in front of him. What is his likely reaction to this?
Valerie	He'd probably say, *"Well, she was lucky that time".*
GP	Yes, he might well say that. What other reaction might he have? Think about how many women there must be driving past him every day without crashing.
Valerie	He might not even notice that she parked well.
GP	Exactly right. So he might discount it by saying she was lucky or he might ignore it altogether. How could you tie in this idea with the negative, self-critical thoughts that you sometimes have about yourself?
Valerie	I can see that I am very quick to notice everything that goes wrong, but I don't always register when things go well or I might discount the good things that I do.
GP	How could you get around this problem? What could you do to make things a little more balanced and fair in the way you see yourself?
Valerie	I could make an effort to notice and remember the things that I do well.
GP	That sounds like a really good idea. How can you make sure that you do remember these things?
Valerie	I suppose I could write them down in a diary.
GP	I would be really interested to see what you find out if you try doing that for a while.

Why do GPs need to know about core beliefs and rules?

When activated, deeper level beliefs can be extremely powerful and are much more difficult to challenge and reframe than automatic thoughts. This can explain why a patient's emotional distress remains high despite using a thought record to evaluate and reframe any automatic negative thoughts. If this is the case, then the next step may be to start working with these more complex and deeply held beliefs.

Working with core beliefs and rules is often time consuming and requires extensive, in-depth therapy which is generally more appropriately carried out during a prolonged course of CBT, rather than in the time-limited setting of a brief GP consultation. Nevertheless, it is important for primary care professionals to understand how deeper level beliefs develop and operate, because:

- Understanding the role of core beliefs and rules gives the clinician a greater depth of understanding and insight into an individual patient's reactions and behaviour.
- The presence of deep-rooted beliefs may explain why methods of reframing negative thoughts have proved unhelpful in certain patients. This may suggest the need for referral to specialist services.
- Identifying the GP's own personal rules may be valuable for understanding our own negative emotional reactions to work-related and personal difficulties.

Maintaining emotional safety

Deeply held, negative core beliefs can be extremely powerful and, when activated, can stimulate a great deal of unpleasant emotion. In order to maintain emotional safety, it is important for health professionals to be sensitive to any cues that suggest the patient is experiencing emotional discomfort, and express empathy for this distress. Try to avoid disagreeing or arguing with patients about the 'best' or 'right' beliefs to hold. Remember that the patient is likely to have held these kinds of belief for many years. Such beliefs may be unhelpful but they may also seem familiar and 'safe' and it can be very threatening to face an entirely new way to view the world.

Identifying core beliefs and rules

Core beliefs and rules may become apparent from particular, recurring themes that arise and result in emotional distress. For example, a person may experience recurrent anxiety in relation to any event with a risk of potential 'failure'.

Another way to identify rules and core beliefs is to ask patients directly about the impact of their early life experiences:

> *"What conclusions did you draw about yourself or others, based on your early experiences in life?"*

> *"How might this influence the problems you are experiencing right now?"*

Core beliefs and rules can also be identified using the *downward arrow* technique. Instead of accepting thoughts at face value, this involves peeling away the layers of thoughts, beliefs and meaning to find out what lies beneath the patient's automatic negative thoughts and fears. This is equivalent to digging up the roots of a weed. The aim is to gently question the basis for any negative thoughts (*Box 10.1*).

Box 10.1	**Questions for the 'downward arrow' technique**

- *"If that thought were true, what would it mean about you?"*
- *"What's so bad about that?"*
- *"What does this situation say about you? What's the worst part about that?"*

Case Example 10.3: Downward arrow technique

Dr T has been a GP for three years. He recently completed a diploma in diabetes management. He has been asked to run a workshop for a group of local GP colleagues on diabetes. The prospect of this presentation fills Dr T with dread. He has always hated giving talks to colleagues. He immediately starts to worry

> *Maybe I don't know enough about the subject to give a talk to all these experienced GPs*
> *What if they don't agree with me or ask me questions that I can't answer?*
> *I would look really foolish*
> *What if I get so nervous I can't get my point across?*

Dr T decides to discuss his fears about making the presentation with a mentor and they agree that it might be helpful to identify any underlying 'rules' which might explain his reaction.

Dr T   When I think about giving the presentation, I get very anxious. I start thinking, *What right do I have to speak to all these experienced GPs?* and *What if they ask me something that I don't know the answer to?*

Mentor   If that really did happen, if they asked you something that you didn't know the answer to, what would that mean about you?

Dr T   Well, I might just stand there, looking really foolish…

Mentor   And if that happened, what would that mean?

Dr T   It would show that I wasn't fully in control. I wasn't prepared enough.

Mentor   What would be the worst bit about that?

Dr T   It would show that I don't really know what I'm talking about. I'm not as much of an expert as they might expect.

Mentor   And if that were true…?

Dr T   I'd be shown up as being incompetent.

Mentor I see. Has this kind of belief come up with you before? Is there some kind of rule that you hold about this?

Dr T I guess that I sometimes feel a bit of a fake. I get really anxious if I think people might 'find me out'.

Mentor And they might find out that…?

Dr T That I don't really know what I'm doing, that I'm incompetent.

Mentor Let's try to work out the exact wording of this rule. For most people it is an 'if…then…' or a 'should…' statement.

Dr T "If I don't always appear completely in control, then people will realise I'm incompetent"

From *theory* to *practice*…

What particular situations do you associate with your own 'heartsink' responses? Think of a recent example. What automatic thoughts arose during that situation?

Now try the 'downward arrow' technique to try to identify what unhelpful rules might underlie your response.

Ask yourself: *'If these negative thoughts are really true, what does that mean about me…?'*

Changing unhelpful rules

Simply identifying and clarifying the unspoken rules that guide people's behaviour can help some patients to begin to undermine and change their unhelpful rules.

Some rules are examples of 'unhelpful thinking styles'. For example, perfectionist beliefs are usually examples of black and white thinking and could be reframed as a 'shades of grey' approach (see *Chapter 6*).

Changing unhelpful rules involves looking for a wide range of evidence both for and against it being accurate or realistic. Rules have usually been held for a long time and the collection of evidence should reflect this. It is also helpful to include a cost–benefit analysis of holding the rule. The final step is to identify an alternative, more balanced rule. This should be a more realistic perspective which retains the advantages of the old rule, while avoiding some of the disadvantages.

Include an assessment of the level of belief in each particular rule ("*How much do you believe this rule, from 0 to 100?*"). The aim is not to eliminate the rule entirely, but to reduce the level of belief in it so that it exerts a less powerful effect over people's lives.

Box 10.2

Evaluating rules and generating helpful alternatives

Evidence 'for' the old rule	Evidence 'against' the rule
"What is the evidence that this rule is accurate or correct? What experiences in your life have proved it to you?" *"What are the advantages of this rule? Are there any ways that it helps you to achieve your goals?"* *"What past experiences might have contributed to the development of this rule?"*	*"What is the evidence against this rule?"* *"Have you had any experiences which contradict it or which show that it is inaccurate or untrue?"* *"Is the rule unfair or unrealistic in any way?"* *"What are the disadvantages of this rule? How does it cause problems for you?"*

Generating a balanced alternative rule:

"What could be a more helpful and realistic alternative to this rule? How could you maintain the advantages of the rule whilst minimising the disadvantages?"

Case Example 10.4: Evaluating rules and generating helpful alternatives

Dr O is a GP who prides herself on having good relationships with her patients. She feels particularly stressed and anxious after seeing Nigel, a 45 year old man with chronic fatigue syndrome. He can be demanding and critical of his care from the practice staff.

He presents to the surgery one day, and insists upon a neurology referral, which Dr O is unwilling to comply with. The result is a somewhat confrontational consultation, and Nigel leaves the surgery angrily. Dr O feels anxious and low. She identifies the following negative automatic thoughts:

> I didn't manage the situation well enough
> I didn't communicate with him very well
> I made a complete mess of this

Dr O realises that she often feels anxious and low if she feels that she has made a mistake or not 'performed' well enough. To identify her underlying rules, Dr O asks herself:

> "If these thoughts were true, what would it mean about me?"
> "What does this situation say about me? What's the worst part about that?"

Using the downward arrow technique, Dr O identifies the following underlying rule: *I must do everything perfectly; otherwise it means that I'm a complete failure.*

Dr O fills out the following chart, to evaluate this rule:

Old rule:	
I must do everything perfectly; otherwise it means that I'm a complete failure	
Evidence *for* this belief	**Evidence *against* this belief**
At school and medical school, it was very important to do well. In childhood, my mother used to get upset if I failed an exam or didn't achieve very high marks. There could be a very serious implication from making a mistake as a doctor. Other people may think less of me if I make mistakes or appear imperfect. There is now a 'blame culture' in the media – making a mistake is viewed as unforgivable. Patient expectations are very high and litigation may follow if I make a mistake. It feels great when I do well. This rule helps me to succeed in life – it drives me on to work hard and do well.	Doing well is not the same as absolute perfection, which is probably impossible to achieve. My colleague, Dr E, makes occasional mistakes but I still think he is a very good doctor and patients really like him. Many successful people fail in some areas of their lives. It's unrealistic to blanket all mistakes together – there are many different degrees. I have made plenty of minor mistakes throughout my life and most did not lead to major disaster. The most important thing is to learn from mistakes rather than label myself as a total failure. I would never be this harsh on anyone else. Everyone makes mistakes sometimes – it is normal and human. My mother got upset when I didn't do well because she loved me and wanted the best for me. She didn't think I was a failure.
New rule:	
It is important to work hard at being 'good enough', but making small mistakes or not being completely perfect is normal and human.	

From *theory* to *practice*…	Think back to your own personal rule that you identified during the previous 'From *theory* to *practice*' reflective exercise.
	Work through the process of gathering evidence for and against the rule. Remember to include a cost–benefit analysis of the rule.
	What could be a more helpful rule? How could you begin to implement this rule in your daily life?
	What would you do differently if you believed this new, alternative rule completely? Can you behave 'as if' the new rule is true?

Using behavioural experiments to overcome unhelpful rules

One of the most powerful ways of altering unhelpful rules is to devise behavioural experiments that reinforce more balanced, helpful rules (*Box 10.3*).

Box 10.3	**Examples of useful behavioural experiments**			
	Unhelpful rule	**Behaviour associated with rule**	**New rule to test**	**Ideas for experiments**
	I must always be in control.	Avoid situations where feel out of control. Behave in a dominant or aggressive manner with others to try to keep control of situations.	It is impossible to be in control of everyone and everything. It is often helpful to allow other people to take some responsibility.	Try participating in situations without trying to take control. Notice what happens to stress levels and reactions from others.
	If I don't please others at all times then they will reject me.	Put others first at all times and ignore own needs.	I deserve to spend some time meeting my own needs as well as those of other people.	Try putting aside some time in the week for enjoyable activities. Learn to say 'no' when necessary. Observe impact on self and others.

Unhelpful rule	Behaviour associated with rule	New rule to test	Ideas for experiments
If I don't try then I can't fail.	Avoid challenges and opportunities. Make little effort to achieve goals.	Trying new things is the only way to make achievements. It's not a disaster if things don't go as I wish. Avoiding things means I will miss out on many opportunities.	Try out learning a new skill or aiming towards a new, positive goal.
If I avoid others then they will never find out how awful I am really.	Avoid contact with other people. Become withdrawn and isolated.	Other people may like me if I give them the opportunity to get to know me better.	Gradually test out having more contact with other people. Try talking and interacting more with others and see what happens.

Once the overall aim of the experiment has been identified, it is helpful to plan out a series of smaller steps to test out in practice (*Box 10.4*).

Box 10.4

Testing out unhelpful rules with behavioural experiments

Old rule: *I must do everything perfectly; otherwise it means that I'm a complete failure.*

The following behavioural experiments show two different ways to test out and reframe this unhelpful rule.

First new rule to test: *Making a small mistake doesn't cancel out all my good achievements.*

What could I do to test if this rule is really true? (what, where, when…?)	Make a list of my achievements. Then make a list of things that I have not done perfectly or mistakes I have made and what happened afterwards. I could then check to see if the mistakes completely outweigh the achievements and if they resulted in major disaster for me.

What do I predict will happen?	I will realise how important it is to avoid mistakes, because I will remember all the terrible things that happened when I made mistakes.
What problems might arise with this plan?	It might make me feel anxious and stressed to think about any mistakes I have ever made.
How could these problems be overcome?	Make sure I spend plenty of time listing achievements before thinking of mistakes.
What happened when I tried the experiment?	*I found that I had made plenty of mistakes in my life, but most of them had no major long-term problems. Some things, which seemed to be problems at the time, actually worked out for the better in the long run.*

What have I learned from this experiment? What is the new, more helpful rule?

It really isn't always a disaster if things don't go completely perfectly. This happens often in life, and usually the problems are overcome in the end.

Second new rule to test: *I will still be 'good enough' if I work less hard and keep time for enjoyable activities.*

What could I do to test if this rule is really true? (what, where, when…?)	Stop working at weekends for three weeks. Plan enjoyable activities instead. Then check with a work colleague about my work performance.
What do I predict will happen?	I won't achieve enough and colleagues will complain about me.
What problems might arise with this plan?	If an important project arises with a deadline that I have to meet urgently.
How could these problems be overcome?	Try to prioritise my work and get the most important jobs done during the week. As a last resort, work on Sunday afternoon if urgent deadline for Monday.
What happened when I tried the experiment?	*I didn't need to work at the weekend. I got most of my work done during the week. My work colleagues had not noticed any change in my overall performance but had noticed I seemed more relaxed and happy.*

> **What have I learned from this experiment? What is the new, more helpful rule?**
>
> *I can still be good at my job even if I don't spend all my weekends working. I am also a lot happier if I make time in my life for enjoyable activities as well as just working.*

Changing core beliefs

As described above, core beliefs are absolutist, black and white beliefs about the self, others or the world. Changing core beliefs is a very long process, because they were usually learned in early life and have been reaffirmed by gathering evidence over a long period of time. It may take weeks, months or even years to gather enough data to counteract a negative core belief by looking for small experiences that support a more positive belief about the self or others.

The new core belief should be a more realistic and fair view of the world, rather than an equally unrealistic positive belief. For example, the negative core belief *'I'm worthless'* might be more helpfully reframed as *'I am good enough'* or *'I have plenty of worth as a person.'*

To slowly shift a core belief, an individual patient needs to keep track of as much evidence as possible that contradicts the old belief and supports the new one. This should include evidence from the past, as well as continuing to monitor for positive events, perhaps using a journal to record the data.

Box 10.5

Questions for developing new core beliefs

- *"What small things have happened in your past to counteract this belief?"*
- *"Are you ignoring or discounting any positive events which might support a more positive view of things?"*
- *"Can you keep an eye out for any small situations that might contradict this negative belief and support the more positive view?"*

Key learning points

- Core beliefs and rules represent deep-seated beliefs, which develop through early and significant life experiences.
- They can be viewed as a system of 'roots' which underlie negative automatic thoughts and can be used to predict emotional distress in specific situations.
- Core beliefs and rules are viewed as *dysfunctional* when they are no longer fully applicable to people's ongoing life circumstances and exert a negative or unhelpful impact on people's lives.
- By behaving 'as if' negative rules and core beliefs are absolute fact, they often become reinforced in reality.
- Being aware of the presence of these beliefs in themselves and others can help GPs to understand and support patients more effectively.
- The presence of active dysfunctional core beliefs and rules can explain why changing automatic negative thoughts is sometimes unhelpful in alleviating a patient's emotional distress.
- Changing these types of belief is a long and slow process, which may be difficult in primary care settings.
- Most individuals with significant problems associated with unhelpful core beliefs and rules are likely to need referral to specialist psychological services. However, some simple primary care strategies that can be helpful alongside a referral include:
  - carrying out behavioural experiments and behaviour change methods to practise more helpful methods of coping with challenging situations
  - keeping a daily diary of information and events that contradict the negative rule or core belief (a 'positive diary').

Chapter 11

Mindfulness and acceptance

What is mindfulness?

Mindfulness represents the ability to stand back and observe our internal processes such as thoughts, emotions and physical sensations. It is a form of self-awareness training that is based on the practice of meditation. It is not dependent on any particular system of belief or ideology.

Mindfulness helps us to disentangle ourselves from our busy minds. We are often not fully aware of mental processes such as thoughts, memories, reflections and judgements about the world, which are guiding and influencing our responses to events (*Box 11.1*). But by being wrapped up in a chain of thoughts, we are less able to cope with situations effectively. Aspects of mindfulness include:

- paying attention to the present moment with an attitude of openness, interest and compassion
- observing our inner experiences, without judging or trying to change or control even distressing or negative thoughts, emotions or physical sensations
- engaging fully in what we are doing rather than getting 'lost' in our thoughts.

Box 11.1	**Explaining mindfulness: automatic pilot**

In a car, we can sometimes drive for miles on 'automatic pilot', without really being aware of what we are doing. In the same way, we may not really be 'present', moment by moment, for much of our lives. We can often be 'miles away' without knowing it.

When on automatic pilot, we are less able to make choices about the best way to cope with a particular situation. We are likely to react to events around us without thinking – often using old habits of thinking and behaviour that may be unhelpful and lead to worsening mood.

By becoming more aware of our thoughts, feelings, and body sensations, from moment to moment, we give ourselves the possibility of greater freedom and choice. We do not have to fall into the same old 'mental ruts' that may have caused problems in the past.

Mindfulness also helps to develop our capacity to experience painful or distressing emotions, thoughts and physical sensations, and to allow them to come and go without battling with them (see also *Box 11.2*). Viewing these experiences from a different perspective can make them seem less threatening or unbearable and allows us to make wiser decisions about how to react to certain situations and ultimately to live a more fulfilling life.

Box 11.2	**Mindful breathing exercise**

- Sit comfortably, with your eyes closed and your back fairly straight.
- Bring your attention to your breathing.
- Notice the sensations in your abdomen as each breath rises and falls. Follow the whole breath all the way in and out like a wave and notice the small pause between each in and out breath. Notice how each breath flows through your whole body.
- You may find that thoughts come into your mind and your attention wanders away from your breathing. The aim is to give any thoughts the space to come and go without getting caught up in the content or judging yourself for having them. If you find yourself caught up in a thought, then simply recognise that this has happened (for example, say to yourself, "*I am thinking*") and then gently bring your focus back to your breathing.
- You may also become aware of sounds, physical feelings or emotions. Again, simply notice and accept these sensations and any reaction that arises in you because of them, and then gently bring your attention back to your breathing.
- Practice this exercise for 5 to 15 minutes each day for at least a week and discover how it feels to spend some time each day just being with your breath without having to do anything more.

Approaches to mindfulness

Mindfulness has been developed and evaluated as two practical techniques: mindfulness-based stress reduction (MBSR) (Kabat-Zinn, 1990) and mindfulness-based cognitive therapy (MBCT) (Segal *et al.*, 2001). There is increasing evidence that both approaches are beneficial for a range of problems, including managing stress, anxiety, depression, and coping with a variety of physical disorders including chronic pain, fibromyalgia and cancer (Kabat-Zinn *et al.*, 1986, 1992, 1998). MBCT has been shown to be an effective treatment for prevention of relapse in depression in people who have been clinically depressed three or more times (NICE, 2009a).

Standard mindfulness training typically involves an 8 week group programme with weekly sessions of around 2 hours and an all-day session in the last week. Sessions involve practising mindfulness exercises such as body scanning, focusing attention on breathing, mindful activities such as walking or movement and practising being fully aware during everyday activities by using breathing as an anchor for attention.

However, more brief practices are still able to help increase mindfulness through the day in bite-sized pieces which can still be very effective in helping to manage difficult emotions or physical sensations.

Acceptance and commitment therapy

Acceptance and commitment therapy (ACT – pronounced as the word 'act'), is one of the recent mindfulness-based therapies that has been shown to be effective with a range of clinical conditions including depression, stress, chronic pain and cancer (Harris, 2006).

The goal of ACT is to create a meaningful life, whilst accepting the pain that inevitably goes along with it. The aim is *not* to attempt to reduce distressing symptoms but instead to tolerate and cope better with symptoms (although this may achieve symptom reduction as a 'by-product' of the process). ACT involves taking effective action to achieve goals in valued life areas, whilst using mindfulness skills to cope with any unpleasant or distressing internal experiences (e.g. negative thoughts, emotions or physical sensations) that may form barriers to these actions.

ACT defines four aspects of mindfulness: acceptance, cognitive defusion, contact with the present moment and the observing self. The aim is to improve 'psychological flexibility' using six core processes (see *Box 11.3*).

Box 11.3	**Core processes of ACT**

- Being in contact with the present moment: awareness and being fully engaged in what we are doing in the here and now.
- Acceptance: allowing thoughts and feelings to come and go without struggling with them or giving them undue attention.
- The observer self: taking a 'big picture' view of the self, differentiating the self from our thoughts or feelings.
- Cognitive defusion: being able to step back and observe thoughts as transient internal events rather than viewing them as absolute fact or threatening experiences.
- Values: clarifying what is significant or meaningful to us as individuals, defining what sort of person we wish to be in our life.
- Taking committed action towards living a valued life: setting goals guided by our values and taking effective action to achieve them.

Experiential avoidance

We may spend a great deal of time and energy attempting to avoid or get rid of unpleasant internal experiences. These 'emotional control strategies' might include:

- withdrawal from socialising in depression to avoid negative thoughts about being boring and worthless
- avoiding specific situations to prevent distressing feelings of anxiety or panic
- carrying out mental rituals or compulsive behaviours in OCD to prevent anxiety
- drinking excessive alcohol or binge eating to avoid distressing feelings associated with low self-esteem
- internal strategies aimed at controlling negative thoughts or emotions such as thinking positively, telling ourselves to 'get over it', or relaxation techniques.

These strategies may reduce negative experiences in the short term but are generally ineffective and can sometimes be costly and self-destructive in the long term. ACT teaches individuals to use mindfulness and acceptance strategies as an alternative to experiential avoidance (*Box 11.4*).

Box 11.4

Letting go of emotional control: the monster and the rope metaphor (Hayes *et al.*, 1999)

Imagine that you are standing next to a wide bottomless pit. On the opposite side of the pit stands a monster. The monster is made up of all of the thoughts and feelings that you fear and avoid. All of your worries, fears, pain and anger are held within this big, dark monster.

The monster is holding a long rope and you are holding onto the other end of the rope. You are engaged in a bitter tug-of-war. You are terrified that if the monster wins, you will be pulled into the bottomless pit. So you dig in your heels, tighten your grip and pull with all your might. This is an effort to control your negative thoughts and emotions. But it is exhausting, and the harder you pull, the stronger the monster seems to become.

Suddenly, you decide to try something different. You let go of the rope and let it fall to the ground. You are aware that the monster and the pit are both still there. But you are no longer struggling and you are no longer afraid of being pulled into the pit. This is letting go of emotional control.

Developing mindfulness

Being in contact with the present moment

Developing mindfulness begins by getting in contact with our own experience in the present moment, in a gentle and non-judgemental way. This includes the mindful breathing exercise (see *Box 11.2*).

Mindfulness is a practical skill, which takes time and practice to develop. However, the practice does not have to be complicated and there are many simple methods of bringing mindfulness into daily life. Even spending just 30 seconds on practice can still be useful. Some brief mindfulness exercises are described in *Boxes 11.5* and *11.6*.

Box 11.5	**The 3-minute mindfulness exercise**

The following exercise is a simple and quick way to step out of 'auto-pilot' and connect with the present moment. Try it whenever you find yourself under pressure or in need of stress relief. Even a few seconds of mindfulness may help to manage stress and tension.

- Sit upright in your chair, adopting an erect posture. Close your eyes and ask yourself, *"What is going on inside me at the moment?"*
- Notice whatever thoughts, feelings and physical sensations are present. Simply acknowledge and accept these, even if unpleasant, rather than trying to change them. It may be helpful to label difficult thoughts or emotions, e.g. *"Feeling anxious"* or *"Thinking about seeing Mrs Smith next week"*.
- Stay with your thoughts and emotions for a few moments and then gently bring your focus to your breathing. Follow each inhalation and exhalation as they flow rhythmically from one to the next. If your mind wanders, gently bring it back to your breathing as soon as you notice.
- Finally, expand your awareness to include your entire body. Notice your posture, facial expression and any physical sensations that are present.
- Now open your eyes. You may feel more settled and calm as you continue your day.

Acceptance

Acceptance involves reducing the struggle to get rid of difficult thoughts and feelings. Trying to push away unpleasant internal experiences creates a mental struggle, which may actually *increase* negative feelings such as anxiety and tension. In contrast, mindfulness creates a mental 'space', which can often help to calm an overactive mind, resulting in a sense of freedom and peacefulness.

| Box 11.6 | **Bringing mindfulness into everyday situations** |

Most daily activities can be carried out mindfully, such as taking a shower, brushing your teeth or doing the washing up. When you take a shower mindfully, try to be aware of the physical actions of rubbing soap into your body or shampoo into your hair. Notice the sensation of the water hitting your skin and how it changes as you move. Bring your awareness to how you are feeling emotionally – are you energetic, sleepy, unhappy or excited? What thoughts or physical sensations are associated with these feelings? Try to just notice the thoughts and feelings rather than getting caught up in them.

Eating mindfully can be a surprisingly enjoyable experience. Try sitting quietly and maintaining awareness whilst you eat, rather than focusing on distractions such as talking, reading or watching TV. Notice what your food looks and smells like. Observe the physical sensations of biting, chewing and swallowing and notice the subtle variations in taste, texture and temperature of the food. If you get caught up in a chain of thoughts, simply bring your attention back to eating as soon as you notice.

Increased acceptance (see *Box 11.7*) makes it easier to take action in valued life directions, rather than getting pulled into an unhelpful cycle of behaviour based on experiential avoidance.

Cognitive defusion

If we are over-attached or 'fused' to a particular thought (e.g. I am a bad person), then we view it as absolute truth and it can exert a powerful influence on our emotions and behaviour. Cognitive defusion allows us to recognise that our thoughts are just words and pictures that float through our minds. It involves noticing thoughts and allowing them to come and go (see *Box 11.8*), rather than becoming caught up in them or holding on to them.

Simple strategies for encouraging cognitive defusion by health professionals include:

- Reflecting back patient's thoughts and worries using language that labels these experiences as cognitive processes rather than engaging with the content of the thought.
  Switch from: "*There's really nothing to worry about*".
  To: "*I notice that your mind is throwing up a lot of worry thoughts here*".

- Trying not to engage, confront or argue with a patient's negative or unhelpful thoughts. For example, a patient may say, "*Taking antidepressant medication is a failure...*"
  Switch from: "*It's not a failure. Plenty of people get depressed and need medication*".
  To: "*Your mind is telling you that taking medication means you have*

Box 11.7

Mindfulness and acceptance of emotions and physical sensations

Next time you experience a strong feeling, emotion or physical sensation, take a few moments to explore it mindfully:

- Start by bringing your awareness to your breathing. Follow a few breaths as they flow in and out of your body.
- Now bring your attention to the feeling or physical sensation that is present. Try to name it: 'pain', 'anger', 'sadness', etc.
- Accept the feeling. Allow it to be present without judging it, resisting or struggling to get rid of it.
- Explore the feeling with a sense of gentle curiosity. How intense is the feeling? Where is it located in your body? Does this feeling have a shape, a texture or even a colour? Is there any tension or change in posture or facial expression?
- Is the feeling static or does it change from moment to moment? What effect does watching the feeling have on it?
- What thoughts or reactions can you notice? Is there an urge to resist or get rid of the feeling? Try to non-judgementally watch this urge and notice how this feels in your body. Allow any thoughts to come into your mind and pass back out again without engaging with them, believing them or arguing with them. It may be helpful to label thoughts ("*Thinking about...*"). Just notice and then bring your attention back to the breath and to the awareness of the feeling in your body.
- What other aspects of your experience can you notice? Spend a few moments discovering any other feelings and sensations that are also present. Include all your senses (hearing, vision, touch, smell).

Box 11.8

Clouds in the sky exercise

Sit quietly with your eyes closed. Imagine that you are lying on your back in a warm meadow, watching white clouds gently floating above you in the sky.

Gently bring your attention to your breathing and then start to notice the thoughts that come into your mind. As you notice each thought, imagine pinning those words or images onto a cloud as it floats past in the sky. Put each thought that you notice onto a cloud, and watch it drift past and eventually disappear. There is no need to make the clouds move faster or slower or to try to change the thoughts in any way.

It is normal for your attention to wander sometimes, so don't worry if this happens. As soon as you notice, just gently bring your focus back onto the thoughts and placing them on the clouds. After a few minutes, bring your attention back to your breath for a moment and open your eyes once more.

failed. I've noticed that your mind has thrown up a lot of negative thoughts recently. How helpful do you think it is to listen to your mind when it is being negative in this way...?"

Some additional techniques for cognitive defusion are shown in *Box 11.9*.

Box 11.9	**Cognitive defusion techniques**

- Labelling your thoughts: switch from *"I'm a loser"* to *"I'm having the thought that I'm a loser"*.
- Labelling emotions and physical sensations: *"I'm having the feeling of ... (describe the feeling)"* or *"I'm having the body sensation of ... (describe the sensation)"*.
- Repeat the difficult thought aloud many times until it becomes a meaningless sound.
- Say thoughts using silly voices (e.g. Donald Duck) or repeat them very slowly.
- Sing your thoughts.
- Watch your thoughts come and go: view your thoughts as leaves floating on a stream or clouds in the sky (see *Box 11.8*); write them on 'post-it' notes.
- Treat "The Mind" as a separate event or person (*"'My Mind' is telling me that I won't enjoy the party"*).
- See negative thoughts as unwanted 'pop up' adverts on the internet.
- Describe the distinction between thoughts that just occur and thoughts that are believed (*"Right now I am believing the thought that I'm bad..."*).
- Ask yourself, how has believing this worked out for me in the past? Is my mind being my friend right now? Is it better to be guided by my mind or by past experience?

Finding the observer self

The process of watching ourselves in mindfulness assumes that there is an 'observer' who is separate from the emotions, thoughts and sensations that are being watched (*Box 11.10*). This helps us to step back from distressing internal experiences rather than being defined or enveloped by them. Instead, we become aware that there are also many other aspects of our experience which continue to exist despite the negative feelings.

Box 11.10

Finding the observing self: the chessboard metaphor

Imagine that your thoughts, physical feelings and emotions are chess pieces on a chessboard. Think of the white pieces as being the thoughts and feelings you would like to have (e.g. happiness, confidence and a sense of wellbeing) and the black pieces as being those that you don't want (e.g. fear, shame, depression or pain).

Imagine that there has been a long chess game, going on for many years, with the two sides battling one another, representing your struggles to overcome your difficult emotions. We tend to feel that the only solution is for one side to 'win' the game. But this is a battle that we hold against ourselves and it may be impossible to 'win' without a heavy cost to ourselves.

Instead, try to let go of the fight and find a broader perspective as your observer self. Picture yourself as the chessboard itself rather than as any individual chess pieces. The chessboard holds the pieces, but it is not equal to the pieces. Similarly, you hold your difficult thoughts and emotions, but you are not equivalent to those thoughts. You can allow the game to continue without being defined by it.

Commitment and action towards living a values-based life

An essential stage in the ACT approach is to set goals for behaviour change based on an individual's core values and meaningful life directions and to then take effective action to achieve them. The aim is to live a life that is consistent with our core values, even if this may mean making space for difficult emotions or physical sensations (see *Box 11.11*).

Some useful questions to identify values and goals include:
- What sort of person is it important for you to be?
- What do you want your life to stand for?
- What would you like people to say about you at your funeral?
- What actions do you need to take that are consistent with these values?
- Can you be willing to take these actions even if it means making room for your [anxiety]?

Setting values-based goals is covered in more detail in *Chapter 8*.

More mindfulness exercises

Many people find it helpful to build a regular mindfulness practice lasting from 10 to 30 minutes into their daily routine. This helps to build the skill of

| Box 11.11 | **Taking life in valued directions: the driving the bus metaphor** |

Imagine you are the driver of a bus. You want to take your bus across town following its designated route. At the first bus stop, you see some passengers waiting so you stop and let them on. But these are not very pleasant passengers. Their names are 'anxiety', 'anger' and 'pain'.

As soon as these unruly passengers get on, they begin to walk up and down the aisle, shouting and causing trouble. They insist that you do not drive across town as planned, but instead take them in a different direction. To stop them causing trouble, you comply, but you discover after a while that you are driving further and further away from the direction that you really wanted to go.

After a while, you get fed up and stop the bus to try to get the troublemakers off. They resist and there is a big struggle. You are not strong enough to make them leave and now the bus is not even moving at all!

Finally, you decide that enough is enough. You tell the passengers that you understand their concerns but that from now on, you will be deciding where to drive the bus. They continue to complain and shout but you carry on driving and just ignore them. Eventually, these difficult passengers sit down and accept that you will be taking the bus in the direction of your own choice.

mindfulness and makes it easier to apply during times of emotional or physical distress. Nevertheless, cultivating even a few moments of mindfulness, perhaps whilst walking or at night before dropping off to sleep, can still be extremely beneficial.

Boxes 11.12 and *11.13* give some examples of alternative mindfulness exercises. It may also be helpful to practise guided mindfulness meditation using an CD or audio recording.

| Box 11.12 | **Mindful walking** |

Mindful walking is one of the easiest forms of mindfulness to fit into a busy, modern lifestyle. People may find it hard to find the time to sit down and focus on their breathing, but most people walk somewhere during the day, even if just for a few minutes. Walking also gives the added opportunity of keeping both mind and body healthy.

- You can practise mindful walking for a few minutes or during a long walk. It can be done in any location, indoors or outside. You can walk slowly or briskly. The aim is to keep a normal gait and simply observe your body as you walk.

Box 11.12
Continued

- Start by taking a few breaths and noticing the breath rising through your body.
- As you walk, move your attention to the sensations as your feet hit the ground. Try to notice every small movement as each foot is placed on the ground and then lifts off again. Notice the feel of the ground beneath your feet or shoes.
- You can stay with your feet or move your attention to other parts of the body. Notice the process of moving your legs, hips, back, arms and chest. Which muscles tense or relax as you move?
- Expand your awareness to notice your surroundings. As you walk, what do you see, smell, hear, taste, and feel? How does the air feel on your skin? What do you notice around you?
- Try to non-judgementally observe any thoughts or emotions that are present as you walk. If you get caught up in thoughts then simply bring your awareness back to the present moment as soon as you notice.
- As you come to the end of the walk, if you have time, take a moment to notice the changes in your body as you stop moving. How are you feeling now, emotionally and physically? Take a moment to reflect on the effects of the exercise before moving on with your day.

Box 11.13

Body scan

A body scan is a mindfulness exercise which many people find relaxing and can be carried out at bedtime prior to sleep. However, the purpose is not to relax but to build awareness and acceptance of the body at the present moment.

- Sit or lie down in a comfortable position. Take a few moments to breathe deeply and allow any tension to flow out of the body.
- Close your eyes and bring your focus to the present moment and your body. Notice the pressure of your body on the bed or ground and allow your body to sink downwards into the surface.
- Move your attention to your feet and toes, both on the surface and deep inside. What do you notice? Are there any physical sensations? If there is any tension or tightness then you could let go and allow the muscles to relax.
- When ready, take your attention up to your lower legs and then upper legs. Each time, notice any sensations that are present. Notice any tightness of the muscles and gently release it.
- Move your attention slowly up your body to your buttocks, waist and lower tummy. Move on to your sides and back.

Box 11.13
Continued

- Slowly move your attention to your chest, shoulders and arms, and then hands.
- Finally move your attention to your neck, jaw, ears, eyes and scalp.
- It may help your focus to keep a light attention on your breathing as you move to each part of the body, and to notice how each breath affects your entire body.
- Finish by taking a few more deep breaths and taking your awareness to your body as a whole. Notice how you are feeling at the end of this exercise.

Tips:

A quick body scan can be carried out either lying or seated, and can be completed in a minute or even 30 seconds. For a brief scan, try to notice large sections of the body at a time (e.g. the whole leg as one section). A longer body scan can take up to 30 minutes and involves focusing on smaller parts of the body (e.g. each finger individually).

Key learning points

- Mindfulness involves paying attention to the present moment and becoming fully aware of our internal processes, without judging, analysing or trying to change them.
- This awareness is carried out with an attitude of gentle curiosity, self-compassion and kindness for any difficult or distressing thoughts, emotions or physical sensations that may arise.
- There are many different mindfulness exercises. It can be helpful to try a range of different approaches to discover which ones are most useful and practical to carry out on a regular basis. They include:
  - mindfulness of breathing
  - mindful walking or other forms of exercise such as yoga and swimming
  - body scanning
  - paying attention to daily activities such as eating, taking a shower or listening to music
- It can be very beneficial to establish a regular mindfulness practice lasting up to 30 minutes once or twice a day. However, even a few moments of mindfulness can be helpful, particularly if carried out on a regular basis.
- You might find it helpful to find a way to remind yourself to be mindful each day. This might be by setting a reminder in your phone

or diary (I will take a one-minute mindfulness break three times a day) or by setting a regular mindful activity (I will be mindful on the walk to work or in the shower every morning).

- Using mindfulness to cope with a difficult situation.
  - By maintaining awareness of our inner reactions when faced by a challenging situation, mindfulness allows us to make wiser choices about how to respond according to our personal values, rather than making a 'knee-jerk' response that may be unhelpful and lead to a downward spiral of negative consequences.
  - Next time you are feeling tense or stressed, take a moment to inwardly reflect and become mindful of what is going on inside you. Give labels to any thoughts or emotions that may be present (*"I am feeling angry"*, *"I'm having the thought that..."*, *"I'm having the urge to yell..."*). Maintain awareness of these inner experiences without struggling or trying to get rid of them, whilst remembering that you do not have to act out any impulses that may be unhelpful. Try not to get so caught up in your inner experience that you view your thoughts as absolute fact. Finally, take a few breaths and decide how best to approach the situation.

Chapter 12

Depression

Understanding depression

Depression is common. Between 5 and 10% of people seen in primary care suffer from major depression, and as many as 2–3 times more people experience depressive symptoms but do not meet diagnostic criteria (see *Box 12.1*) for major depressive disorder (Katon & Schulberg, 1992).

Box 12.1	**Diagnosis of major depression (DSM-IV Criteria: APA, 1994)**

Five of the following criteria (including at least one of the first two criteria) must have been present *almost every day for more than two weeks*, and must cause significant impairment in social, occupational or other areas of functioning.

- Depressed mood for most of the day
- Reduced pleasure or interest in usual activities for most of the day
- Fatigue or loss of energy
- Substantial change in appetite or unintentional weight loss or gain
- Insomnia or hypersomnia
- Psychomotor agitation or retardation
- Diminished ability to think or concentrate, or indecisiveness
- Feelings of excessive guilt or worthlessness
- Recurrent thoughts of death or suicide

Cognitive-behavioural therapy for depression

CBT is the psychological treatment of choice for depression (NICE, 2009a). It is as effective as antidepressant drug therapy for major depression in primary care (Scott *et al.*, 1997). It also has a lower rate of long-term relapse than antidepressants (Paykel *et al.*, 1999), because patients develop lasting skills to help them cope with difficulties in life. In severe depression, a combination of CBT and antidepressants is more effective than either treatment alone.

A combined approach to depression for primary care

NICE advocates a stepped care approach to depression management, which includes psychological approaches and medication as potential treatment options in the primary care setting (*Box 12.2*).

Brief CBT approaches by primary care health professionals are particularly useful for patients with mild depression, for whom there is little evidence that antidepressant medication is effective. This can be carried out alongside self-help strategies, graded exercise programmes or medication if appropriate.

Box 12.2

Stepped care model (NICE, 2009a)

Focus of the intervention	Nature of the intervention
Step 1 All known and suspected presentations of depression	Assessment, support, psycho-education, active monitoring and referral for further assessment and interventions
Step 2 Persistent sub-threshold depressive symptoms; mild to moderate depression	Low-intensity psychological and psychosocial interventions, medication and referral for further assessment and interventions
Step 3 Persistent sub-threshold depressive symptoms or mild to moderate depression with inadequate response to initial interventions; moderate and severe depression	Medication, high-intensity psychological interventions, combined treatments, collaborative care and referral for further assessment and interventions
Step 4 Severe and complex depression; risk to life; severe self-neglect	Medication, high-intensity psychological interventions, electroconvulsive therapy, crisis service, combined treatments, multiprofessional and inpatient care

Understanding depression

Typical thoughts and thinking styles in depression

Depressed people characteristically develop *negative* thinking patterns, which are often examples of *unhelpful thinking styles* (*Box 12.3*).

Box 12.3

Common unhelpful thinking styles in depression

- Black and white thinking (*"I am completely useless"*)
- Negative, self-critical view of self (*"I am such an idiot"*)
- Ignoring positives (*"Nothing went well this week"*)
- Mind-reading (*"He thought I was boring"*)
- Negative view of the future (*"Nothing will ever get any better"*) and predicting catastrophes
- Taking excessive personal responsibility / self-blame (*"I ruined the party for everyone"*)

Depressed people tend to have self-critical and self-blaming thoughts, which lower confidence, self-esteem and cause problems in relationships with others:

"I'm a terrible parent; I'm a burden to others; I'm useless"

These thoughts are usually *self-fulfilling* because thinking so negatively tends to prevent people from behaving in constructive or positive ways.

Depressed people also take a negative and pessimistic view of the world. They jump to the worst conclusions and perceive others as critical, uncaring or hurtful. For example, they may focus on one minor criticism whilst ignoring a barrage of compliments.

"The world is so full of terrible events; Nothing ever goes right for me"

Negative thinking or hopelessness about the future is common in depression, and at its most severe, can be linked with suicidal thoughts and behaviour.

"I'll never get a job – what's the point in trying?"

"I will never get over this depression. Nothing will get any better"

From *theory* to *practice*...

Notice the negative thoughts displayed by depressed people. Look for negative thoughts about the self, world and future. Which unhelpful thinking styles are most common?

At this stage, do not attempt to *challenge* these thoughts. When you notice a negative thought, try pointing it out to the patient and empathise with the distress that the thought might cause (*"It must be very difficult to think that way..."*) Then discuss the impact of thinking so negatively (*"I wonder how it affects your mood to think that way...?"*).

> **Case Example 12.1: Negative thoughts in depression**
>
> Cathy is a 26 year old bank clerk who suffers from mild depression. Here, she describes a barbecue that she attended at the weekend.
>
> *"I went to Alison's barbecue at the weekend. I didn't want to go, because I knew that I wouldn't enjoy it. I never have anything interesting to say. While I was there I made a terrible mistake – I forgot the name of Alison's sister, Joanne. I've only met her once before and my mind went blank. I looked like a complete fool. I tried to make it up to her by apologising and asking about her children, but I don't think that was enough. Alison will never invite me to another party."*
>
> Read through the text and identify Cathy's negative or unhelpful thoughts.
>
> **Negative, unhelpful thoughts:**
> *"I won't enjoy the barbecue"*
> *"I never have anything interesting to say"*
> *"I made a terrible mistake by forgetting Joanne's name"*
> *"I looked like a complete fool"*
> *"It wasn't enough to apologise and ask about her children"*
> *"Alison won't invite me to any more parties"*
>
> Which unhelpful thinking styles are represented by these thoughts? (See Box 12.3 for a reminder.)

Feelings and emotions in depression

Depressed people experience a wide variety of negative emotions, including:
- persistent depressed mood – feeling sad, low, bleak, numb and empty
- loss of enjoyment or pleasure in usual activities
- anxiety, worry and panic
- anger and irritability: with self and others
- guilt and shame.

Biological factors and physical symptoms in depression

Depression is associated with a wide range of unpleasant physical feelings and symptoms. Many depressed people present to health professionals with physical or somatic rather than psychological symptoms (NICE, 2009a). Common physical reactions include the following.
- *Low energy and lethargy*: feeling tired all the time is one of the most common physical aspects of depression. It often results in a marked reduction of activity which worsens mood and fatigue as a vicious cycle.

- *Disturbed sleep:* includes difficulty getting off to sleep, early morning wakening or excessive sleeping.
- *Difficulty concentrating and problems with short-term memory:* people may find it difficult to read or follow a TV programme or conversation.
- *Changes in appetite and weight:* may be weight loss or weight gain due to 'comfort eating.'
- *Reduced libido:* loss of interest in sex.
- *Becoming 'slowed up'* (*psycho-motor retardation*): people often think and move more slowly than usual. This may include other bodily functions such as becoming constipated.
- *Physical agitation:* muscular tension and restlessness.
- *Increased pain:* people often feel pain more intensely when depressed.
- *Associated physical conditions:* depression is more common in people with physical health conditions.

From *theory* to *practice*…	Remember to ask depressed people about any physical symptoms, including low energy and fatigue. Explain that these are caused by the patient's depression and that they are likely to improve with treatment for depression.

Altered behaviour in depression

Unhelpful behaviour plays a key role in exacerbating or maintaining feelings of depression. This includes reduced activity and increasing unhelpful activities.

Reduced activity

Depressed people withdraw from social activity and reduce participation in enjoyable activities, such as hobbies and interests. They may also reduce activities that give life a sense of meaning or achievement, such as taking exercise, going to work, or daily activities like household chores. In more severe depression, people stop caring for themselves adequately.

These changes in behaviour may be due to:
- lethargy and tiredness (*"I'm too tired to do it"*)
- depressed mood and lack of enjoyment in usual activities (*"There's no point in going because I won't enjoy myself"*)
- negative thinking and low motivation (*"I can't be bothered to try"*).

Reducing activity only worsens depression as a vicious cycle. Becoming withdrawn and reducing enjoyable activities makes life increasingly mundane and isolated. Avoiding routine tasks and chores, such as ironing or washing up, can make people feel ashamed and guilty, and increases their sense of failure and lack of worth (*"I can't even manage to keep the house tidy – I'm completely useless"*).

Increasing unhelpful activities

Depressed patients may also develop new, unhelpful behaviours, which make their problems worse, including:

- misuse of alcohol or drugs
- self-harm
- making excessive demands or seeking reassurance from others
- sabotaging their own attempts to achieve positive goals ('setting themselves up to fail')
- behaving in ways which increase the likelihood of being let down or rejected by others.

From *theory* to *practice*...	Ask depressed patients whether they are behaving differently: *"What do you do differently, now that you feel so depressed? How did you behave before you felt depressed?"* Is this behaviour helpful or unhelpful? How does it affect their depressed feelings?

The role of environmental and social factors in depression

Life events, social difficulties and environmental problems, both past and present, all contribute to the development of depression (*Box 12.4*).

Box 12.4	**Risk factors for depression**
	• Female sex: women are twice as likely to develop depression, particularly if caring for young children and lacking social support • Socioeconomic factors such as financial problems, poor housing or unemployment • Family history of depression • Loss of a parent before adolescence • Lack of social support network (e.g. close friends or family) • Negative or stressful life events • Experiencing chronic physical illness or being a carer

Vicious cycles in depression

Negative thoughts and low mood in depression tend to reinforce one another as a vicious cycle.

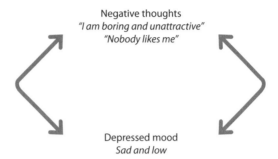

Similarly, reducing activity and withdrawing from other people also tends to make depression worse. This makes the person feel even more isolated and confirms any negative beliefs about their own lack of self-worth.

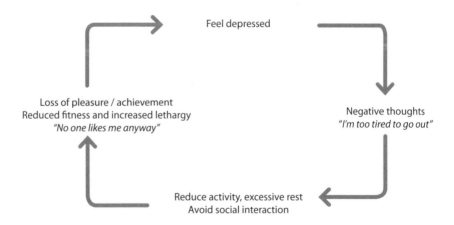

From *theory* to *practice*...	Remember to gather information about all five areas of the CBM when assessing depressed patients. Make particular note of any unhelpful behaviour such as reducing activity.
	Can you identify any vicious cycles? What behavioural changes might enable the patient to break these cycles and make small steps forwards?

Case Example 12.2: Using the CBM to understand depressed patients

Roger is a 40 year old teacher who became more depressed 6 months ago when he was having problems with a colleague at work. He started antidepressant medication, which did improve his mood and had few side-effects. However, he still periodically feels low and depressed. He does not want to change his medication.

Roger's GP asked Roger to identify a specific situation that illustrated his difficulties and together they created the following CBM chart:

Problem list:
1. Anxiety and lack of confidence to speak up during staff meetings
2. Not managing to get jobs such as marking or lesson planning done on time
3. Feeling tired and lethargic
4. Irritable and snappy with wife and children

Roger chose to focus on not managing to get jobs such as marking or lesson planning done on time

Specific situation that illustrates the problem: Tuesday evening, coming home from school and realising there is huge amount of marking to do.

Thoughts	Feelings
"I won't ever be able to cope with this workload – there's too much to do"	Depressed
"I will just make a mess of it"	Down
"I haven't achieved anything this evening"	Fed up
"I'm a terrible teacher"	

Behaviour	Physical symptoms
Puts off starting the work	Tired and sluggish
Dozes in front of the TV all evening	Sleepy and exhausted

Environment / situation / other problems

Works as English teacher in a secondary school

Married to Valerie, two children, good relationship, but he feels increasingly irritable with small problems that arise in the family

Problems last year with a difficult head of department – little confidence in own work

---

Reflection

What vicious cycles can you identify for Roger? What 'handover' questions could the GP ask that might help highlight these to Roger?

Using 10 Minute CBT with depressed patients

Depressed people often welcome a psychological approach to their problems. Nevertheless, symptoms such as tiredness, lethargy, difficulty concentrating and a continual barrage of negative thoughts make it difficult for depressed people to actively engage in the approach. Some key consultation skills that can help patients overcome these difficulties are shown in *Box 12.5*.

Box 12.5

Key consultation skills to use with depression

- *Written information*: providing written self-help leaflets and a summary of any discussion is especially important in depression where patients have poor concentration and memory.
- *Focus on specific, concrete examples*: ask the patient to choose the most important issue to discuss. Often the discussion can be generalised to other areas of the patient's life.
- *Guided discovery*: encourage patients to take the lead in discussions and discover new perspectives for situations themselves. Remember that depressed people may think slowly and have difficulty concentrating. Keep questions simple and allow them time to come up with answers.
- *Homework*: encourage the patient to make real changes in their life based on your discussion. Focus on increasing activity levels. Remember to review homework when you next see the patient.

Empowering explanations in depression

An important aim for GPs is to help patients understand depression better. Try to use the five areas of the CBM to map out and explain the vicious cycles that typically maintain depression. Always ask a handover question to encourage the patient to reflect on your discussion:

> *"What do you make of all this information that we have gathered? How could you use this approach to help you improve things?"*

The most important empowering explanation for depression involves discussing *depression tiredness*. Depressed people commonly feel tired and lethargic, and consequently rest and reduce activity even more. However, the tiredness associated with depression is *made worse* by rest and the most helpful and effective way to increase energy and reduce tiredness in depression is to *increase activity*, which energises people and improves mood.

> **From *theory* to *practice*…**
>
> Ask patients whether tiredness is preventing them from increasing their activity levels. If so, does rest seems to make them feel less tired? Explain that 'depression tiredness' is made worse by rest but can be improved by gradually increasing activity levels to build fitness and muscle strength.
>
> Then try to collaboratively agree some goals to increase activity levels in bite-sized steps. If the patient is unsure, you could plan a behavioural experiment to test out the impact of increasing activity by rating their feelings of lethargy before and after various activities.

Making behavioural changes in depression

Depressed patients benefit from increasing activity levels *despite* their negative thoughts or feelings, including lethargy or tiredness. Regular aerobic exercise may be as effective as antidepressants in improving mood in depressed patients (Babyak *et al.*, 2000).

Increasing activity has several useful effects:
- enjoyable activities make life more pleasurable and interesting
- participating in activities distracts people from continually mulling over negative thoughts that worsen mood
- success at even small tasks like tidying the house or washing the car gives patients a sense of achievement and increased control over their life
- increasing exercise may directly alter brain biochemistry, promote positive feelings and improve mood.

Encourage the patient to **behave 'as if'** they are no longer depressed. This involves making positive behavioural changes *despite* feeling tired or lethargic. Choosing small, achievable goals will help build patients' self-confidence and self-esteem.

Initially, the patient may not enjoy activities as much as before being depressed. The first step is to restart the activities anyway. Participating in events can still increase patients' sense of achievement. Over time, the increase in activity will help the depression to lift and allow the enjoyment to slowly return.

> **Case Example 12.3: Changing behaviour in depression**
>
> *George has been depressed for over 2 years. He feels tired and lethargic and tends to take naps during the day. "I'm too tired to do anything right now. I need to rest for a while." George's GP suggests that he could try a behavioural experiment to test out whether these thoughts are accurate.*

They decide to compare two different ways of coping when he feels tired. On one day, he will go to bed and sleep as soon as he feels tired. On the next day, he will go for a 10 minute walk instead. He will do this on alternate days until he next sees his GP. George agrees to rate his feelings of sadness and lethargy before and after each strategy.

On the next appointment, George reported that he had been surprised to find that resting usually made him feel *worse* rather than better – his mood dropped lower and he usually felt even more tired. However, doing activity had actually lifted his mood on several occasions. He had also achieved several jobs that he had been putting off for some weeks, and felt a sense of positive achievement from this.

After the experiment, George reframed his original thought: "Resting when I am tired usually makes me feel worse, it is usually better to try to do something more active" and agreed to continue to gradually increase his activity levels further.

Behavioural activation in depression

Behavioural activation is an extremely effective strategy for overcoming depression (see *Chapter 7*). The first step is for the patient to keep track of their current behaviour using a behaviour monitoring form (*Figure 12.1*). They should keep track of what they do throughout the day and rate each activity according to its importance and enjoyment. Daily completion of the monitoring form is an essential part of this approach.

Monitoring behaviour can highlight unhelpful behaviour patterns where patients are spending a lot of time on activities that are neither enjoyable nor important. It may also help to identify any positive or helpful activities and encourage the patient to continue these.

After monitoring for several weeks, the next step is to begin to plan new activities. It is useful to set goals according to the individual patient's values and important life areas (*Chapter 8*). Encourage patients to aim for small, realistic increases in meaningful and enjoyable activities, keeping in mind the principles of pacing and avoiding boom–bust activity patterns that worsen fitness over time.

The patient can write their goals onto a daily monitoring form using a different colour. Then, they complete the daily monitoring form as usual, and compare what they planned with what they actually achieved. If the patient did not achieve their planned goal then consider setting a more achievable goal or helping the patient to find ways to overcome the obstacle next time.

Time	Activities (give details)	Importance (rate 1–10)	Enjoyment (rate 1–10)
06:00–07:00 am			
07:00–08:00 am			
08:00–09:00 am			
09:00–10:00 am			
10:00–11:00 am			
11:00–12:00 am			
12:00–1:00 pm			
1:00–2:00 pm			
2:00–3:00 pm			
3:00–4:00 pm			
4:00–5:00 pm			
5:00–6:00 pm			
6:00–7:00 pm			
7:00–8:00 pm			
8:00–9:00 pm			
9:00–10:00 pm			
10:00–11:00 pm			
11:00–12:00 pm			
12:00–02:00 am			
02:00–04:00 am			
04:00–06:00 am			

Figure 12.1: Behavioural monitoring form

Case Example 12.4: Using an activity chart in depression

Penny has been depressed for 9 months. She feels low, tired and has very little motivation to carry out her usual tasks. Penny's GP suggested that she could use a behavioural monitoring form to keep track of her activities throughout each day. They spent a few minutes during the appointment filling in the chart for that day, to give Penny some practice at using the chart. She also agreed to continue filling in a daily chart at home for the next 2 weeks.

Time	Activities (give details)	Importance (rate 1–10)	Enjoyment (rate 1–10)
07:00–08:00 am	Got up and got kids ready for school. Felt irritable and shouted at kids.	8	4
08:00–09:00 am	Had breakfast and did school run.	9	6
09:00–10:00 am	Came home feeling tired. Watched TV.	5	5
10:00–11:00 am	I wanted to do some housework but still tired. Carried on watching TV.	2	3
11:00–12:00	Got up and did the washing up. Did a few household jobs.	5	3
12:00–1:00 pm	Had lunch. Still hungry after so had a bar of chocolate.	5	4
1:00–2:00 pm	Went to supermarket and bumped into a friend. Bought myself a magazine.	7	7
2:00–3:00 pm	Came to visit GP to talk about how I'm feeling.	8	5

Two weeks later, Penny and her GP talked through some of her completed charts. Penny was surprised that she often achieved more than she had expected through the day. But it was also clear that she was spending more time on activities such as watching TV even though this was not rated as important or particularly enjoyable.

Penny's GP pointed out that there seemed to be very few enjoyable or social activities in her week. Penny agreed that she had cut down on many activities which she had previously found enjoyable – such as physical exercise and seeing friends.

The next step was to plan some important life areas and set some activity goals. Penny decided that her important life areas were relationships with friends and hobbies. She planned to make time to meet a friend for lunch and to start swimming again.

Physical exercise

Physical exercise has a direct effect on mood to alleviate depression, and is therefore a particularly important activity for the patient to carry out. This could include walks with friends, gardening, swimming or playing with children. Walking is a particularly accessible option, which is cheap and does not necessarily involve a great deal of time. Even a very short walk (5–10 minutes) can be very beneficial to alleviate depressed feelings.

Coping with negative thoughts in depression

The process of *identifying* and *labelling* negative thoughts helps to strengthen the view that such thoughts are simply *opinions* rather than absolute facts and helps to promote a more balanced and realistic perspective.

Distraction

Distraction is a simple but effective short-term strategy to reduce the number and impact of negative thoughts by focusing the mind elsewhere. Concentrating on a practical activity or exercise can distract a depressed person from their negative thoughts and lift their mood.

Exploring and reframing negative thoughts

As always, the first stage is to identify any negative thoughts that arise during a specific situation. Ask the patient to choose one negative thought to look at in more depth. The next step is to try to identify evidence both for and against this thought and finish by asking the patient to try to find an alternative, balanced perspective.

Mindfulness

Mindfulness-based cognitive therapy has been shown to reduce relapses in patients with recurrent depression (NICE, 2009a). Practising mindfulness can help people to see more clearly the patterns of thoughts in the mind and to recognise when their mood is beginning to go down, enabling them to take action at an early stage to prevent further decline. It also helps the person to focus on the present moment, rather than getting caught up in negative thoughts about the past or the future which serve to lower mood.

Key learning points

Summary of the cognitive behavioural model for depression:

Thoughts / thinking styles	Feelings
• Negative thoughts: self-criticism, negative view of world, hopelessness about future • Low motivation and apathy • *"I'm useless. I'm a failure"* • *"I'm a terrible parent. It's all my fault"* • *"Nothing will get any better"*	• Sadness, low mood, loss of enjoyment • Anxiety and worry • Guilt, shame, anger
Behaviour	**Physical symptoms**
• Reduce meaningful and enjoyable activities, excessive rest • Withdrawal and loss of social interaction • Other unhelpful activities, e.g. misuse of alcohol, self-harm, reassurance-seeking	• Low energy and tiredness, poor sleep • Poor concentration and memory • Changes in appetite and weight • Loss of libido; ill-health
Environment / social factors	
• Lack of social support, unemployment, financial problems, stressful life events • Loss of a parent before adolescence, family history of depression	

- 10 minute CBT strategies are particularly useful for GPs to help patients with mild to moderate depression. The approach can be combined with self-help, graded exercise and antidepressant medication.
- Increasing meaningful and enjoyable activity is one of the most important methods of breaking the vicious cycles that maintain depression.
- Use principles of behavioural activation to encourage your patients to be more active *despite* negative thoughts or feelings of lethargy. By behaving 'as if' they are less depressed, they are likely to feel better.
- Encourage patients to set their own behavioural goals based on their personal values and important life directions. To build confidence, make sure these goals are bite-sized and easily achievable. Where possible, encourage social interaction and social support for maintaining the goals.

Chapter 13

Insomnia

What is insomnia?

Insomnia is an inability to sleep. As many as 1 in 5 adults do not get as much sleep as they would like. Insomnia includes a range of sleep disturbances including:

- difficulty getting to sleep
- waking frequently in the night
- waking early in the morning and being unable to get back to sleep
- feeling tired or not refreshed by sleep.

The occasional night of missed sleep will cause little harm, but persistent insomnia can be a very distressing problem with a major impact on daytime wellbeing and functioning. Consequences of insomnia include daytime sleepiness, difficulty concentrating, problems making decisions, poor performance in daily activities and altered relationships with others. It is particularly dangerous for people who drive or operate heavy machinery.

People who suffer from insomnia may become low or depressed. However, insomnia may also be a presenting feature for a disorder such as depression, anxiety or dementia. Lack of sleep can also increase the risk of high blood pressure, obesity and diabetes.

What are the normal stages of sleep?

Normal sleep is divided into three different stages.

- Rapid eye movement (REM) sleep comes and goes throughout the night and is the stage during which most dreams occur. The brain is very active during REM sleep, but the body is relaxed, apart from the eyes, which flick rapidly from side to side.
- Quiet (non-REM) sleep. There are four levels of quiet sleep that involve increasing depths of sleep. The brain is quiet but the body may move around. The deepest stages are known as deep sleep.
- Short periods of waking for 1–2 minutes. It is normal to have several short periods of waking throughout the night. These occur about every 2 hours, but become more frequent towards the end of the night. Because they are only short, we don't normally remember these. We are more likely to remember them if we feel anxious or there is something else that disturbs the sleep such as noise or physical discomfort.

How much sleep do we really need?

Most adults need around 7–8 hours of sleep per night, but this varies widely between different individuals, with some needing as little as 3–4 hours per night and others needing up to 10–12 hours. The amount required can depend on many factors including age and activity levels. Babies and young children need much more sleep than adults. The amount of sleep that adults need generally reduces with age, often by several hours per night.

The important thing is to get enough sleep to feel refreshed and active during the day, without being too drowsy or tired. Some people worry that they are not getting sufficient sleep when in fact they feel fine during the day and have no need for any more sleep. The short wakeful periods through the night can also sometimes seem longer than they really are and contribute to a perception of insomnia that is not really accurate.

Causes of insomnia

Many factors can contribute to the development and maintenance of insomnia. It is helpful to look at these in terms of the five areas of the CBM.

Background factors, life events and the physical environment

Stressful life events such as bereavement, exam stresses, work deadlines and financial problems can cause sleeping difficulties. People may have difficulty relaxing at bedtime and lie awake worrying about these problems. Physical factors in the bedroom such as having an uncomfortable mattress, curtains that allow the light through, being too hot or cold, a partner who snores or a noisy TV in the next room can also interfere with sleep.

Physical problems and medication

Physical conditions such as pain, itching, difficulty breathing, coughing, restless legs or needing to go to the toilet during the night can all lead to difficulty sleeping. Some drugs also interfere with sleep (see *Box 13.1*), including caffeine which is found in coffee, tea, cola drinks, hot chocolate, some herbal drinks and many cold remedies and headache tablets. Taking regular caffeine to overcome daytime sleepiness can be addictive and leads to a vicious cycle of increased insomnia and tiredness over time.

Alcohol tends to make people fall asleep quickly but generally leads to broken, unrefreshing sleep and increased daytime tiredness. Heavy alcohol intake causes depression and anxiety which also interfere with sleep.

Box 13.1	**Drugs which can cause insomnia**

- Alcohol
- Caffeine
- Antidepressants
- Decongestants
- Beta-blockers
- Thyroid hormones (particularly if the dose is higher than needed)
- Corticosteroids
- Sleeping tablets may cause a rebound insomnia when stopped
- Some illegal drugs have a stimulant effect on the body

Thoughts and thinking styles

Anxious or worry thoughts can interfere with sleep. These may be general worries about life problems as well as worries about the lack of sleep itself. People may 'catastrophise' the risk and consequences of not sleeping:

> *"I'll never cope at work tomorrow. I'll be exhausted. The day will be a disaster."*

> *"This lack of sleep will cause me serious physical harm."*

This anxiety about sleep leads to increased tension and wakefulness and reduces sleep still further in a vicious cycle. Thoughts predicting poor sleep are also generally self-fulfilling:

> *"I'll never sleep tonight! It will be such an awful night!"*

Feelings and emotions

Many different emotions are associated with sleeping difficulties. These include anxiety, depression, irritability, anger, shame and guilt.

Unhelpful behaviour

A number of behaviour patterns can exacerbate sleeping difficulties, including the following:

- Poor preparation for sleep with no relaxing bedtime routine. It is particularly unhelpful to carry out physically or mentally stimulating activities just before bed.
- Using the bedroom for activities other than sleeping, such as reading, working or watching TV. This makes people associate the bedroom with wakefulness and worsens sleep.
- Unhelpful sleep patterns such as going to bed particularly early or late at night, getting up late in the morning, and having daytime naps. These interfere with the sleep–wake cycle and worsen insomnia.

- Going to bed when not feeling sleepy.
- Lying awake in bed for long periods of time, worrying about not being asleep.
- Having woken in the night, carrying out unhelpful activities such as working or watching a scary movie.
- Repeatedly checking the clock to see what time it is and how much sleep has been missed.

From *theory* to *practice*…	Give an empowering explanation to a patient who worries about catching up with missed sleep.
	Many people who have difficulty sleeping worry about how to catch up with all the sleep that they missed. However, it is only necessary to catch up on about one-third of any sleep missed. After missing a night of sleep, we will experience a deeper and more refreshing sleep afterwards, which enables us to catch up with the missed sleep more quickly.

Case Example 13.1: Insomnia

Kelly is a 45 year old woman who visits her GP complaining of insomnia. This has been going on for around 6 months. Kelly is currently going through a divorce. She has two children aged 7 and 9 and is worried about how they will cope with the change. She has a busy and unpredictable job working as a self-employed beautician. She says that she does not feel depressed but is exhausted and fed up with her lack of sleep.

Kelly's GP completes a five areas assessment of her problems using the CBM:

Specific recent example: Last night I was lying in bed and couldn't get to sleep. I couldn't drop off to sleep for a couple of hours and woke several times in the night. I was shattered in the morning.	
Thoughts	**Feelings**
"I really need to get to sleep. I'm going to be exhausted again tomorrow."	Fed up and low
"How will I get through the day?"	Worried and anxious
"I'm worried I'll have a breakdown if I carry on like this."	Frustrated
Recurrent thoughts and worries about her current life stresses (children, divorce, etc.)	

Behaviour	Physical problems
Active evenings – she often has late clients or goes to the gym after the children are in bed	Exhausted
	Difficulty concentrating at work, making silly mistakes
She drinks strong coffee or diet cola to get through the day and usually has several glasses of wine in the evening	Headaches and back pain
She gets up at a regular time each morning	
She goes to bed at around 11pm but finds it difficult to drop off and lies in bed for several hours; sometimes she watches TV in the bedroom or reads a magazine	
Environment and background	
Going through a divorce, worried about the children	
Self-employed beautician – busy and unpredictable – some financial worries	

Management of insomnia

Sleep hygiene

Sleep hygiene involves a range of advice and tips for promoting better sleep, including behavioural, environmental and lifestyle factors (*Box 13.2*).

Box 13.2

General advice for improving sleep ('sleep hygiene')

- Get up at the same time every day, 7 days a week, even if you feel you have not had enough sleep. This will gradually train your body to sleep at night.
- Avoid all daytime naps, no matter how tired you feel during the day.
- Only go to bed when you feel sleepy tired. The usual signs include yawning, a lack of energy, heavy eyes and an involuntary tendency to nod off.
- If you don't fall asleep after 15 minutes, go to another room and do something relaxing. Return to bed when you are sleepy tired. If the same thing happens, simply get up a second time.
- Use your bed only for sleep or sex. Don't read, watch TV, make phone calls or work in bed.
- Develop a regular 'wind-down' routine starting 60–90 minutes before bedtime. This includes stopping activities that stimulate the mind and doing relaxing activities such as a warm bath, reading or gentle stretching each night.

Box 13.2
Continued

- Exercise during the day will improve your physical health, mood and make you more tired at night. However, avoid vigorous exercise just before bedtime.
- Minimise your caffeine intake and don't drink coffee or tea within six hours of bedtime.
- Cut down your alcohol intake. It causes night-time wakening and increased tiredness the following day.
- Try eating a light carbohydrate snack or drinking a warm milky drink before bed.

Create a good sleeping environment

Ensuring that the bedroom is a restful sleeping environment can help to improve the quality of sleep. Having a comfortable mattress and pillows and appropriate bed covers for the time of year (not too hot or cold) is important. It is helpful to remove excess clutter and reminders of work or other stressful stimuli. Thick blinds, curtains or wearing an eye mask will help to create a dark environment. If noise is a problem, ear plugs can help.

From *theory* to *practice*... Encourage patients with insomnia to only use their bed for sleep. This will help to build the association between the bedroom and successful sleep. Explain that people who do not suffer from insomnia are generally able to read or watch TV in bed without affecting their sleep. This is because they are usually not worrying about falling sleep and are not carrying out these activities in an attempt to make themselves drop off. In contrast, for a patient with insomnia who is extremely worried about getting to sleep, the bed and any activities carried out there become associated with a high level of anxiety. It is important to break this association between the bed and anxiety, so patients with sleeping difficulties should avoid carrying out any other activities whilst in bed.

Using a sleep diary

If difficulty sleeping has become a problem, it can be helpful for patients to keep a 'sleep diary' to measure their sleep patterns over a period of around 2 weeks. This should be completed each morning about the previous day (*Figure 13.1*).

Using a sleep diary to improve sleep efficiency

A key goal for improving insomnia is to improve sleep efficiency. This is the ratio of time spent asleep to the total amount of time spent in bed. Once a sleep

Measuring your sleep pattern	Monday	Tuesday	Wednesday	Thursday	Friday
Did you nap during the day? For how long?					
Did you exercise? For how long?					
How many drinks containing caffeine? How many after 6 pm?					
How much alcohol did you drink?					
What time did you get up this morning?					
What time did you go to bed?					
What time was 'lights out'?					
How long did it take to drop off to sleep (minutes)?					
How many times did you wake during the night?					
What is the longest you were awake for (minutes)?					
How long did you sleep in total (hours/minutes)?					
Did any specific worries or problems keep you awake? What?					
Measuring the quality of your sleep					
How tired did you feel immediately on waking (0–10)? 0 = terrible, 10 = best ever					
How did you feel during most of the day (0–10)? 0 = terrible, 10 = best ever					
Overall sleep quality (0–10)? 0 = terrible, 10 = best ever					

Figure 13.1: Sleep diary

diary has identified current patterns of sleep behaviour, the patient can then begin to improve sleep efficiency using stimulus control and sleep restriction.

Stimulus control

Stimulus control re-establishes the association of the bed and bedroom with sleep, rather than with the frustration and anxiety of trying to sleep. The patient should go to bed only when sleepy, and get up at the same time each day regardless of how much they slept. Most good sleepers will fall asleep within 15 minutes of getting into bed. So, if unable to fall asleep after 15 minutes (without clock-watching), the patient should get up, go to another room and return to bed only when sleepy tired.

Sleep restriction

Sleep restriction limits the time in bed to the amount of time a patient actually normally sleeps. The first step is to use a sleep diary to calculate the average sleep time and then limit the total time in bed to that as a maximum. For example, if a patient sleeps an average of six hours a night, the total time in bed is limited to six hours.

The patient plans their preferred time to get up and then goes to bed six hours before this. They should stick to this routine for a few days. This is likely to make the individual feel a bit more tired and will help to make the sleep more refreshing and uninterrupted. The patient should continue to keep a sleep diary and at the end of each week, if things are improving, they can plan to go to bed 15 minutes earlier. Over the next few weeks they gradually build up the total sleep without allowing it to interfere with the overall sleep efficiency.

Case Example 13.2: Using a sleep diary to improve sleep efficiency

Tracey is a 43 year old woman with a long history of sleeping problems. She has no symptoms to suggest depression or other problems that could be the underlying cause of her insomnia. Her GP asks Tracey to complete a sleep diary to monitor her current sleep pattern.

On returning to the surgery, the diary shows that she goes to bed at 10 pm and watches TV or reads in bed for an hour. She turns out the light at 11 pm but does not fall asleep until at least midnight. She reports very broken sleep and says she is sometimes awake all night. On average she sleeps around 7 hours per night. She usually gets up at 8 am but sometimes stays in bed later if she is very tired. She often feels tired through the day. She sometimes rests on her bed but does not nap.

Using a sleep diary to improve Tracey's sleep efficiency

Tracey's GP encourages her to improve her sleep efficiency using sleep restriction and stimulus control. Her total average sleep is around 7 hours, so they agree that she will go to bed at 1 am – 7 hours before her usual wake up time.

They also agree that if she is unable to fall asleep or return to sleep within 15 minutes, she will get up and go to another room, and only return to bed when sleepy tired. She will continue this pattern until her sleep improves.

By the second day of sleep restriction Tracey is falling asleep more quickly and has much improved sleep efficiency. She continues this for a week and then brings her bedtime back by 15 minutes to 12:45 am. Over the next few weeks, Tracey's sleep continues to improve. However, when her bedtime reaches 11:15pm she finds that her sleep efficiency starts to decline and her sleep becomes poorer. She sets her bedtime 15 minutes later and finds that by going to bed at 11:30 she is able to achieve good sleep on a regular basis.

Managing worry thoughts

Strategies for managing night-time worry thoughts include the following.

Stop trying to sleep

It is extremely helpful for patients with insomnia to adopt a more relaxed and accepting attitude towards sleep. Trying too hard to force sleep to come will have the opposite effect by increasing anxiety and tension about the lack of sleep. Paradoxically, trying *not to sleep* may actually make it easier to drop off.

The patient could try to switch from: *"I must sleep – it's 2.30 am and tomorrow will be a disaster if I'm tired"* to *"I would much prefer to sleep but I can still cope with less sleep, I've done it before"*.

Put the worries aside

It can be helpful for patients to use a diary or a notebook to write about their worries in the early evening. This is similar to the 'worry time' used in generalised anxiety disorder (*Chapter 14*). They should write about their day, any problems or issues that they are facing, as well as anything that may be coming up in the future that may be causing concern. The diary should also include ideas for solving these problems. This process often helps the patient to put their worries aside at night.

If worrying thoughts pop up at night, the patient can think, *"I've already dealt with these worries today and I can think about them again in the morning"*.

The patient could also keep a piece of paper next to the bed to make a note of any new thoughts that arise, which can be dealt with in the morning.

Evaluating unhelpful thoughts

Cognitive strategies for improving insomnia include looking for unhelpful thinking styles and using thought records to identify and challenge negative beliefs about sleep (*Figure 13.2*). It can also be helpful to identify any unhelpful thinking styles such as catastrophic thinking, unrealistic expectations and all-or-nothing thinking.

Negative thought about sleep	Balanced, alternative thought
"I didn't get a wink of sleep all night."	*"I did get some sleep according to the sleep diary, even if it wasn't as much as I'd really like."*
"I can't function without at least 8 hours of sleep."	*"I have been coping without sleep for many months. Perhaps I don't need quite as much sleep as I thought."*
"I should be able to sleep well every night like a normal person. I shouldn't have a problem!"	*"Lots of people struggle with sleep from time to time. I will be able to sleep with practice."*
"I'm never going to be able to sleep well. It's completely out of my control."	*"Insomnia can be cured. If I stop worrying so much and focus on positive solutions, I can beat it."*
"If I don't get some sleep, I'll mess up my presentation and lose my job."	*"I can get through the presentation even if I'm tired. I can still rest and relax tonight, even if I can't sleep."*

Figure 13.2: Reframing negative thoughts about sleep

Problem-solving

Problem-solving strategies can help to reduce the anxiety and stress associated with particular life events and difficulties (see *Chapter 9*).

Meditation and relaxation

Relaxing and enjoyable activities can help to improve sleep by calming the body and mind. This could involve reading a book, taking a bath or listening to relaxing music. Gentle exercise, yoga or stretching can also be helpful. Practising daily relaxation or controlled breathing techniques can also be helpful.

Using mindfulness can also help manage a busy or active mind at night. Rather than becoming involved with the thoughts which make people feel frustrated and tense, it can be helpful to use mindfulness techniques to let go and watch as each thought floats through the mind, allowing it to pass through and disappear. This creates a distance from the thought, and encourages the development of a more peaceful mind, with less struggle and tension within. Mindfulness meditation can also help people to cope with distressing or unpleasant symptoms, such as pain, that may also interfere with sleep. See *Chapter 11* for more details on mindfulness.

Key learning points

Summary of the cognitive behavioural model for insomnia:

Thoughts	Feelings
Preoccupation and worry about the lack of sleep	Anxiety and worry
Catastrophisation about the consequences of not sleeping	Irritability, anger, frustration, guilt
"I'll never get to sleep – I can't cope without 8 hours of sleep each night"	Low mood and depression
"Going without sleep will cause me to have a breakdown"	
Behaviour	**Physical problems and medication**
Poor preparation for sleep; going to bed when not sleepy	Lack of sleep causes fatigue, muscle aches, sleepiness and difficulty concentrating
Stimulating activities in bed (e.g. reading, watching TV)	Physical symptoms such as pain or breathlessness interfere with sleep
Daytime napping or getting up late	
Lying in bed for long periods when awake	Caffeine, alcohol and many medications interfere with sleep
Repeatedly checking the clock	

Environment and background

Stressful life events may trigger sleeping difficulties.

Physical factors such as an uncomfortable bed, being too hot or cold and too much noise or light can interfere with sleep.

- Make a thorough assessment of patients presenting with insomnia to rule out underlying causes such as depression or physical illness which may need to be treated first.
- Ask for a specific recent example of a time that they had difficulty sleeping. Then establish the key thoughts and behaviours that might be contributing to the problem.
- Ask the patient to complete a sleep diary for at least four nights to get a better understanding of their sleeping patterns. This often clearly identifies useful strategies for making change.
- Useful approaches to improving insomnia include:
  - practising 'sleep hygiene' with a regular relaxing bedtime routine
  - increasing daytime exercise and reducing naps
  - stimulus control – only go to bed when sleepy and get up if not asleep within 15–20 minutes
  - sleep restriction – aim to sleep no more than the number of hours that you currently actually sleep and gradually build upwards
  - manage worry thoughts using a daily diary and thought records
  - relaxation and mindfulness.

Chapter 14

Anxiety disorders

Anxiety is an unpleasant emotional state associated with fear and distressing physical symptoms. It is a normal and appropriate response to stress but becomes pathological when the reaction is extreme and disproportionate to the severity of the stress. This chapter provides an overview of several anxiety disorders including panic attacks, generalised anxiety, social anxiety and obsessive compulsive disorder.

Panic disorder

Panic disorder is common – 1 in 10 of the population experiences a panic attack at some point in their life. It is important to exclude other causes of panic symptoms, such as excess caffeine, amphetamines or hyperthyroidism.

The CBT model views panic attacks as *catastrophic misinterpretations of normal bodily symptoms* (Beck *et al.*, 1985; Clark, 1986). The patient experiences harmless, often anxiety-related symptoms, and incorrectly interprets them as indicating imminent disaster, such as a heart attack, suffocation or going mad. The anxiety that develops in response to these fears results in further symptoms, which worsen the patient's anxiety as a vicious cycle.

Key features of panic attacks:
- they come on suddenly and quickly
- they are associated with intense fear and anxiety
- the most intense feelings of panic are short-lived (although the patient may feel anxious to a lesser degree for some time after the most intense feelings have passed).

Thoughts and cognitive factors in panic

In anxiety disorders, people have catastrophic thoughts where they overestimate the risk that something bad will happen and focus on the worst possible outcome of events. They also tend to underestimate their ability to cope if the feared event did take place.

During a panic attack, people generally fear that something terrible is about to happen in the near future. Common thoughts include:

"I am having a heart attack or a stroke"

"I'm going to choke or suffocate"

"I will faint or collapse"

"I am going to lose control"

"I will go mad or crazy"

"I'm going to make a complete fool of myself"

From *theory* to *practice*...	Try asking the patient to describe a recent example of a panic attack. Try to find out what they feared *at the time* of the panic attack by asking: *"What thoughts were going through your mind when you started to feel anxious?"* *"What did you think was happening to you?"* *"What physical symptoms did you notice? What did you think these might be due to?"* *"What is the worst thing that might happen?"* By identifying the patient's specific fears, you will be able to give more effective empowering explanations. This also provides later opportunities to test out the beliefs using thought records or behavioural experiments.

Case Example 14.1: Identifying thoughts associated with anxiety

Linda has been experiencing panic attacks over the past 6 months, and has been avoiding going to busy shops and supermarkets because of her anxiety. In the following dialogue, Linda's GP explores her specific thoughts and fears.

GP	You feel anxious at the thought of going into the supermarket. What is it about this situation that makes you feel so anxious?
Linda	Well, I might not cope with it.
GP	When you say *"I might not cope"* what do you mean by this?
Linda	I might get really anxious.
GP	And what is the worst thing that might happen if you became anxious?
Linda	I would make a fool of myself in front of everyone.
GP	What do you mean by *"make a fool of myself"*? What would you do?
Linda	If I had a panic attack, it would be really embarrassing.
GP	What can you imagine happening during the panic attack that might mean that you made a fool of yourself?
Linda	My mind gets confused and my thoughts race so much during the attack. I get scared that I might start babbling complete nonsense to

> other people. I might lose control and make such a scene that other people will think I am completely crazy. I worry that I could get taken away to a mental hospital.
>
> **GP** That sounds like quite a scary image to have.
>
> **Linda** Yes, it's really terrifying.
>
> **GP** I'm sorry to hear that. The good news is that although anxiety is very unpleasant, it cannot really make you go crazy. Maybe we can talk about your fears and try to make that image a bit less frightening.
>
> **Linda** That would be a huge relief.

Feelings in panic disorder

The commonest feelings in panic disorder are extreme anxiety and intense fear. These usually arise suddenly and are usually relatively short-lived. The feelings are extremely distressing and unpleasant.

Physical symptoms in panic disorder

The physical response to anxiety and panic reflects the adrenaline-based, sympathetic response to fear. This results in a wide variety of powerful and often unpleasant physical symptoms, including:

- rapid heartbeat, palpitations
- rapid breathing (hyperventilation); feeling short of breath
- chest pain
- tightness in the throat, choking sensations
- gastrointestinal symptoms: feeling nauseous, abdominal pains
- feeling faint, dizzy or unsteady; shaking
- numbness and tingling in fingers, toes and lips
- headache, back pain
- sweating and hot flushes
- difficulty concentrating; feelings of unreality

The role of behaviour in panic disorder

During a panic attack, people believe strongly that they are threatened by a serious, imminent danger. Their behavioural reactions, described below, are therefore usually aimed at preventing this harm from occurring.

Avoidance

Patients with panic disorder tend to avoid situations that they associate with anxiety, such as busy shops, confined spaces or giving presentations. This can result in major restrictions in the patient's life and leads to a long-term loss of confidence in their ability to deal with stressful situations, and an increase in anxiety over time.

Escape from 'dangerous' situations

People commonly react to rising feelings of anxiety by *escaping* from anxiety-provoking situations.

Safety behaviours

Safety behaviours represent specific actions that anxious people undertake in an attempt to protect themselves from particular feared outcomes (*Box 14.1*). These behaviours prevent the patient from learning that the feared catastrophe would probably never have happened. Instead, the patient assumes that their behavioural reaction was responsible for keeping them safe (*"If I hadn't left the room at that point then I would have definitely lost control..."*). If the patient remains to face the scary situation, then they are able to learn that no harm would have come to them and develop confidence that they *can* cope without taking any special precautions.

Box 14.1	**Common safety behaviours in panic attacks**

Sensations	Misinterpretation / thought	Safety behaviour
Palpitations, racing heart Chest tightness Sweating	*"I'm dying"* *"I'm having a heart attack"*	Sit down, avoid exertion Take medication (e.g. beta-blockers) Try to slow heart rate Call an ambulance or visit doctor
Breathlessness	*"I'm going to suffocate"* *"I can't breathe"* *"I'm choking"*	Take deep breaths Sit by open windows Go into open air
Unreality Muddled thinking Inability to concentrate	*"I might lose control"* *"I'm going mad"* *"Other people will think I'm crazy"*	Try to keep control of mind Look for exits in public Avoid public areas
Dizziness	*"I'm going to faint or collapse"*	Sit down Hold onto someone Avoid going out alone

From *theory* to *practice*...	Try using the following example to illustrate the unhelpful effect of avoidance behaviour to patients.
	A child believes that a monster lives under her bed. She feels certain that if she were to look under the bed, the monster will leap out and eat her. So, she avoids looking under the bed, and never gets eaten. In the child's mind, this proves that as long as she avoids looking under the bed, she will remain safe.
	How can this child discover that there really is no monster under the bed?

Body scanning and checking

Continual monitoring and focusing on bodily sensations (checking for danger) increases the patient's awareness of normal sensations, which are then interpreted negatively and may trigger the panic cycle.

From *theory* to *practice*...	Use the following experiment to explain the unhelpful effect of concentrating on bodily symptoms to patients:
	Take a few moments to pay attention to your left foot. Notice any sensations, including temperature, pain, aches or any other physical feelings that may be present.
	Ask: *"What sensations did you become aware of? What is the impact of looking for physical feelings?"*
	Most people find that as soon as they begin to look for physical sensations, they become aware of them. Common feelings include tingling, heaviness or discomfort.
	If we are not concerned about the meaning of such sensations, then noticing them is unlikely to result in anxiety.
	Imagine, however, if you noticed tingling in your foot and thought to yourself, *"This must mean that I'm having a stroke"*. This is very likely to lead to feelings of anxiety, which may be further compounded by *normal* physiological reactions to fear, such as hyperventilation, which further increase sensations of tingling or dizziness and reinforce fears about having a stroke.

Triggers for panic attacks

A panic attack usually arises after a particular trigger, which might include:
- having an anxiety-provoking thought or image pop into the mind
- getting anxious about a potentially stressful situation
- becoming aware of physical symptoms related to minor illness

- the effect of drugs, including alcohol or caffeine
- physical exertion causing changes in heart rate and breathing.

Once the patient has experienced a panic attack, they may develop future anxiety about the possibility of having another one. This panic about panic leads to a vicious cycle of increased anxiety and worry.

Vicious cycles in panic disorder

The vicious cycles of panic disorder are illustrated in *Figure 14.1.*

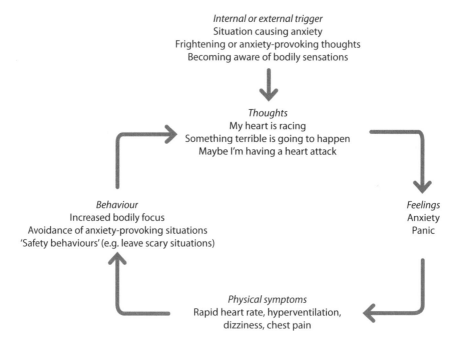

Figure 14.1: CBM of panic – vicious cycles

Giving empowering explanations in panic disorder

Empowering explanations of anxiety

The first step in primary care is to give patients clear and credible explanations for the physical and emotional symptoms that arise during panic attacks. You should acknowledge that the patient's symptoms are real and highly distressing, and go on to explain that these represent normal physiological responses to scary thoughts and situations, rather than being due to a potentially life-threatening condition.

Explaining the fight or flight response

Anxiety responses have evolved over millions of years to protect us from physical danger as part of the 'fight or flight response' and are very useful in the right time and place. The symptoms of panic are not a sign that something is going wrong – they indicate that the body is doing exactly the right thing to prepare for the perceived threat (*Box 14.2*).

Problems arise when the fear response is happening at the wrong time or when it persists beyond the point where it is useful. In the modern world, people rarely face physical threats so these physical preparations made by the body may be unhelpful in many circumstances, but they are ***not*** dangerous.

Box 14.2	**Explaining physical symptoms using the fight or flight response**

Symptom	Empowering explanation
Heart racing, palpitations	Your heart beats faster to get oxygen around the body to provide the fuel that helps your muscles fight or run away to escape the danger. This is essential so that we don't pass out or faint when faced with a dangerous situation.
Chest tightness, feeling short of breath	We breathe faster and deeper when anxious, to get oxygen into our bodies more efficiently. This over-breathing or hyperventilation makes the muscles of our chest wall feel tight. However, we have plenty of oxygen going around the system so there is no risk of suffocation. *Behavioural experiment:* ask the patient to take a deep breath then take another one straight away. Notice how it leads to tightness and discomfort in the chest.
Chest pain	By breathing so hard and working so hard, it can make the muscles of our chest start to ache, just like any other muscle in the body. Because they are so sensitive this pain can feel quite severe but it is not a sign of a serious underlying medical problem.
Dry mouth, difficulty swallowing, choking sensation	When anxious we tend to get a dry mouth. This can make it harder to swallow and lead to uncomfortable sensations that make it feel like we are choking, although this is not actually the case. *Behavioural experiment:* ask the patient to swallow quickly five times in a row and notice what sensations arise. Try it yourself now.
Feeling light-headed and dizzy	When we breathe quickly during anxiety it leads to changes in carbon dioxide levels in the blood, which can make you feel light-headed and dizzy. However, you are highly unlikely to faint or collapse because your blood pressure tends to be higher during a panic attack.

Box 14.2 Continued	Neck/back pain and muscular shaking	Muscles are tensed in preparation to leap quickly into action. This leads to muscular aches, pains and shaking. *Behavioural experiment:* ask the patient to tense their arm for up to a minute. Notice the pain and shaking that arises.
	Difficulty concentrating, poor memory, muddled thoughts	During a panic attack your mind is programmed to be on the alert for danger at all times. This makes it very difficult to focus on one thing and can make it seem like your memory is not so good.

Anxiety is not dangerous

People often hope to eliminate anxiety altogether in order to feel better. However, this is unrealistic and may reinforce the underlying belief that anxiety is dangerous and should be avoided at all costs. It is more helpful to aim to become less worried about anxiety when it does arise. This has the additional benefit of reducing unpleasant anxiety symptoms by breaking the vicious cycles that often maintain and worsen anxiety.

Cognitive strategies to manage panic attacks

Different strategies are helpful at different stages of a panic attack. In the midst of a panic attack it is difficult to think clearly or rationally, so it is difficult to use cognitive restructuring techniques at this point. The patient will need to use strategies such as distraction and controlled breathing to reduce anxiety to more manageable levels before they are able to rationally evaluate the level of danger.

Distraction

Distraction offers a simple way to reduce the impact of anxious thoughts and feelings. Useful techniques include simple puzzles, mental arithmetic, counting or repeating the words of a song in the mind (see *Chapter 6*). Although distraction is a useful short-term strategy for coping with anxiety, it does not help the patient to challenge and overcome their negative thoughts and fears and there is a risk that patients begin to use distraction as a safety behaviour, to avoid facing their fears.

Helping patients to view panic as less dangerous

It is important to emphasise that panic attacks feel very unpleasant but are not really dangerous and will always go away after a short while.

<table>
<tr><td>From theory to practice…</td><td>

Ask the patient to count how many panic attacks they have ever experienced in their life. Be precise by calculating the average number per day or week, over a period of months to years. The total number may be several hundred. Then ask the patient:

"Have you ever actually had a heart attack/gone crazy?"

"Even though you have experienced over 200 panic attacks, nothing has ever actually happened that you really fear. What do you make of this?"

Remember to highlight the fact that the feelings of anxiety always go away in the end. If the patient waits long enough, they will feel better. This can be helpful for patients to remind themselves during episodes of anxiety.

</td></tr>
</table>

Finding evidence for alternative perspectives

A key strategy for managing panic disorder is to reframe the negative thoughts that underlie feelings of anxiety and panic (*"Just because I think I'm having a heart attack doesn't make it true"*). This can decrease anxiety and reduce the likelihood of fear spiralling upwards into a panic attack.

It is useful to look for written evidence for and against the most frightening thoughts using a thought record. Patients may wish to write down this evidence and carry it around as a 'flashcard', which they can read whenever they feel anxious.

Case Example 14.2: Reframing scary thoughts

Peter has been experiencing panic attacks for the past six months. At the peak of his panic attacks he has the following thought: "If I carry on feeling so bad, then I will certainly have a heart attack".

Anxious thought to test out:	
"If I carry on feeling so bad, then I will certainly have a heart attack"	
Evidence *for* the hot thought	Evidence *against* the hot thought
What makes you say that this thought is true?	Is there anything that shows that the thought is not completely accurate?
Has anything happened to prove it to you?	Are there any other ways to view the situation?
Do any past experiences fit this belief?	Is this way of thinking an 'unhelpful thinking style'?
	What would be more realistic?

My heart is racing and I feel sweaty – this is what happens during a heart attack	There are many other reasons for having a racing heart and getting sweaty, e.g. during exercise, and exercise is good for the heart
I get chest pain when I feel very anxious – this could be a sign of strain on the heart	Lots of people experience extreme stress, such as being mugged or being a soldier in battle, but don't all have heart attacks
I saw a TV programme where a very stressed-out, anxious man ended up having a heart attack	The 'fight or flight' anxiety response isn't dangerous – it is a normal reaction to stressful situations
Anxiety makes my blood pressure go up – this is bad for the heart	I have had many panic attacks and nothing bad has ever actually happened
I feel so bad during the attack – it must be something really serious	I had my heart checked by the doctor and they found nothing wrong
	Panic does cause a brief rise in my blood pressure but it is only if blood pressure is constantly raised that it becomes a problem; my blood pressure has been checked and it is normal
	I feel really bad during panic attacks but this doesn't mean that I am having a heart attack; people can still feel very bad, even when there is no danger

Alternative / balanced thought to replace the hot thought

Write an alternative or balanced thought which takes into account evidence for and against the hot thought. Try to be fair and realistic.

"The symptoms that I get during a panic attack are better explained by anxiety than having a heart attack. They feel really bad but are not dangerous and cannot actually hurt me."

Behaviour change in panic disorder

Useful behavioural change techniques for managing panic disorder include changing unhelpful reactions such as avoidance or safety behaviour. You could encourage patients to plan a behavioural experiment to find out what happens when the patient faces their fears or stops using safety behaviours.

Reducing avoidance behaviour

Patients can gradually reduce avoidance behaviour using 'graded practice'. There are several stages for this (Kennerley, 1997).

1. Make a list of situations which the patient is avoiding or that make them anxious. Identify a wide range of situations, including some which are not too challenging or frightening.
2. Ask the patient to rank the situations into order of increasing difficulty.
3. Choose the first situation as a target for the patient to achieve; if it still seems overwhelming, try breaking it down into smaller steps.
4. Plan the strategies for coping with any problems or anxiety that may arise. This might include using distraction, controlled breathing or relaxation strategies.
5. The patient tries out the task. They should repeat it several times, until it no longer seems difficult or anxiety-provoking.

The first step is to complete the task *despite feeling anxious*. By repeating the task several times, their anxiety will naturally reduce over the long term. It can be useful for some patients to work through particularly scary situations in their imagination, before trying in real life. This involves visualising successfully coping with the difficulty, including imagining using specific coping strategies to overcome their fear.

Case Example 14.3: Using graded practice to overcome agoraphobia

Beryl suffers from agoraphobia. She experiences anxiety and panic attacks when away from home, especially in busy or crowded areas. Together, Beryl and her GP create the following list of anxiety-provoking situations, beginning with the least difficult:

1. Go to the local shop with my husband during a quiet time of day
2. Go to the local shop and husband waits outside
3. Go to the local shop alone at a quiet time
4. Go to the local shop at a busy time, buying only one or two items
5. Go to the local shop at a busy time and spending longer there, looking for several items
6. Go to a mini-market with my husband
7. Go to the mini-market alone at a quiet time
8. Go to the mini-market alone at a busy time
9. Go to the supermarket at a quiet time
10. Go to the supermarket at a busy time

Behavioural experiments to elicit feared physical symptoms

Behavioural experiments can be used to elicit feared physical sensations and enable the patient to learn that these symptoms do not necessarily indicate imminent catastrophic danger, for example:

Hyperventilation: breathing deeply and rapidly for a few minutes produces a wide range of sensations, often similar to those experienced during panic. Afterwards, use handover questions to encourage the patient to reflect on this:

- *"Were these symptoms similar to the ones that occur during panic? What do you make of the fact that you can bring them on by breathing quickly for a few minutes?"*
- *"How does this affect the idea that the symptoms mean you are having a heart attack? Can heart attacks be brought on like that?"*
- *"How quickly did the symptoms subside after you stopped breathing fast? What do you make of this?"*

Contraindications to hyperventilation include cardiac problems, high blood pressure, pregnancy and asthma / COPD.

Exercise tasks: some patients avoid exercise due to fears that the associated rapid heart rate or sweating may be dangerous. Challenging these beliefs might involve encouraging the patient to run up steps, skip, walk briskly or go jogging.

Chest pain: ask the patient to take a deep breath and then try to take another deep breath on top of this. This often causes chest discomfort and supports the explanation that chest pain relates to overuse of thoracic muscles during a panic attack.

Physical strategies for reducing panic

Relaxation training can help patients to reduce their background levels of stress and muscular tension, which may reduce the likelihood of developing panic attacks. This could involve yoga, progressive muscular relaxation or meditation.

Controlled breathing techniques can help to avoid hyperventilation during a panic attack. This technique requires practice when patients are feeling calm and relaxed, before they will be able to use it effectively during panic attacks.

From *theory* to *practice*...	Practising controlled breathing: ask the patient to take a slow, deep breath, whilst counting up to four in their mind. Next, they should hold the in-breath, again counting up to four. Then breathe out slowly whilst counting to four. Finally, hold the exhaled breath and again count up to four:

In   1...2...3...4...

Hold   1...2...3...4...

Out   1...2...3...4...

Hold   1...2...3...4...

This process should be repeated until they feel more relaxed and calm. Ideally, the patient should practise this technique for *four minutes*, carrying it out *four times each day*.

Box 14.3	**Summary of self-help strategies for managing panic reactions**

- Remind yourself that the feelings of panic are *normal bodily sensations* related to anxiety and are not harmful. Read through your flashcard of alternative helpful ways to think about the situation.
- Remember that anxiety, whilst extremely unpleasant, is *not really dangerous*. It is a mechanism which has evolved over millions of years to *protect us* by helping us cope with physical danger.
- Try not to run away. Instead, try to accept what is happening to you. If you wait long enough, the fear will pass. This will make it less likely to arise in the future.
- Use coping strategies like distraction or controlled breathing to reduce your unpleasant anxiety symptoms.
- Remember that frightening thoughts are just *thoughts* – they are not necessarily true or accurate. Just because something *seems true* does not mean that it is.
- Try to find more helpful and realistic ways to look at any thoughts that might be making your anxiety worse.
- When you feel better, think back to what triggered off the panic. What kinds of anxious thought were going through your mind at the time?
- Whilst you are feeling calmer, try to find a more balanced or alternative way to look at the situation, which might be less likely to make you panic in future.

Generalised anxiety disorder

Generalised anxiety disorder (GAD) involves persistent 'free-floating' anxiety that arises in a wide range of situations. The anxiety and worry is extremely distressing and is associated with a high level of impairment in daily functioning and disrupts people's work, relationships, hobbies and social activities. It is often a long-term problem, and symptoms should be present on most days for at least 6 months before a diagnosis is made.

Typical features of GAD

Thoughts

Patients with GAD spend a lot of time worrying. It is difficult to control these worry thoughts, which are like a broken record going around and around in the head. They tend to involve many catastrophic and "what if the worst happens....?" thoughts. The level of worry is out of proportion to the risk of the problem actually occurring.

People with GAD often grow fearful of their own anxious thoughts and feelings. This 'worry about worry' leads to increased anxiety and fear as a vicious cycle:

"I can't control the worry. I will go crazy with worry. I'm going to become ill or die because of all this worry."

In some cases, people may also hold positive beliefs about worry as a protective or helpful coping strategy:

"Worry helps me to avoid problems or prevent bad things happening. It helps me to be prepared and get motivated."

However, in GAD worry is unhelpful and involves focusing on worst case scenarios rather than coping strategies. It tends to distract people from coping with problems rather than helping to solve them.

Feelings

Patients with GAD experience chronic anxiety and stress, and may be irritable and easily annoyed. They may also develop secondary low mood and depression.

Physical symptoms

Patients with GAD often feel agitated, on edge, restless and have difficulty concentrating. They may also experience a wide range of other physical symptoms including muscle pain and tension, gastrointestinal symptoms, problems with sleep, palpitations and sweating. In primary care, patients often present with physical symptoms so it is important to specifically ask about worry when patients present with potentially anxiety-related symptoms.

Behaviour

Typical behaviour in GAD includes avoidance of situations that may cause anxiety. This means that they often do not face up to or deal with possible problems, leading to an increased belief in their inability to cope with difficulties and a loss of self-confidence and increased anxiety over time.

Case Example 14.4: Generalised anxiety disorder

Claire is a 52 year old housewife who is married with one grown-up son. She attends the surgery with muscle pains, difficulty sleeping and palpitations. Her investigations are all normal. She often seems anxious during her appointments.

When Claire's GP asks about anxiety symptoms, he discovers that she worries about many different issues. She constantly worries about her son and husband and phones to check on them many times a day. She also worries about her health, "*I always imagine the worst*". Her worries have a huge impact on her life and she's hardly going out or seeing friends. She can't sleep as her mind continually goes over and over her different worries.

CBT approaches to GAD

Worry time

A strategy for reducing the amount of time spent worrying is to plan a specific 'worry time' (e.g. 30 minutes) every day. If the patient feels anxious or begins to worry during the day, they can write down a brief description of the worry in a diary (maximum 3–4 words) and say to themselves, "*I will think about this later at worry time*". Then they continue with daily activities or if necessary, carry out a distraction activity.

During worry time, the patient thinks about all of their worries and concerns for the day. If they don't feel worried at this point, then they do not have to worry! It is also helpful to plan an enjoyable or distracting activity to carry out after worry time is over.

Dealing with 'what if' thoughts

'*What if...?*' thoughts that something terrible is about to happen are common in GAD. The first step is to identify the specific feared outcomes that are being predicted by the patient. This can help an anxious patient:

- recognise that their fears are exaggerated and unlikely to occur
- find ways to prevent the worst outcome from taking place
- plan how to cope with any difficulties if they do arise.

Rather than offering reassurance that the worst will never happen, it is often more helpful for patients to build their confidence in dealing with difficulties by planning how they might cope if feared situations really did arise (*Box 14.4*).

Box 14.4

Coping with feared situations

- How could you cope if this really did happen?
- What skills do you have that might help to deal with this situation?
- What past experiences might help you deal with this?
- What help, advice or support could you obtain from other people?
- What information could you find out that might help you deal with this situation?

Another method of coping with '*what if...?*' thoughts is to construct a '*then what...?*' plan for dealing with particular feared outcomes.

Case Example 14.5: Finding coping strategies for 'what if...?' thoughts

Gabriella is a 25 year old student. She worries a great deal about lots of different problems in her life including many catastrophic and '*what if...?*' thoughts. She is particularly anxious about a job interview next week. Her GP helps her to identify coping strategies for her '*what if...?*' thoughts, using the questions from *Box 14.4*:

'What if...?' thoughts and fears	'Then what...?' coping strategy
"What if my mind goes blank during the interview?"	I could take a deep breath and tell the interviewers that I feel nervous and need a moment to compose myself, and then ask them to repeat the question.
"What if they ask me a question and I can't think of an answer?"	I can practise interviews with my friend Claire. I will read up on the likely questions that they will ask. If I really don't know the answer then I may have to say so – they might help me out.
"What if I say something really stupid?"	I could say to the interviewer, "I think I may not have expressed myself very well, what I meant to say was…" Anyway, it is impossible to be 'perfect' and always say the right thing.

"What if they are really aggressive interviewers?"	I will try not to take them too seriously. I will just answer the questions as best I can. I might not even want to work in an office where people are very aggressive.
"What if I drop something on my smart clothes before the interview?"	I will eat breakfast before I leave home and then not eat anything that could damage my suit once I have left the house. I could also take a wet wipe to clean anything that I spill.
"What if I don't get the job?"	I can see this interview as good practice for other jobs. I will keep applying for jobs until I find the right one.

Overcoming avoidance

Overcoming avoidance behaviour should be planned as a series of graded steps enabling the patient to build confidence in their ability to cope with anxiety-provoking situations.

Develop more positive beliefs about worry

It can be helpful to look for the evidence for and against any beliefs that the patient holds about worry, and then look for more balanced alternative thinking styles (*Box 14.5*).

Box 14.5

Questions to help challenge unhelpful beliefs about worrying

- What makes you think that worry is uncontrollable?
- Has your worry ever stopped because you were interrupted or distracted by something (e.g. by a phone call or someone coming to the front door)?
- What makes you think that worry is dangerous?
- Have you ever actually [gone crazy, had a heart attack...] whilst worrying?
- Do people with highly stressful jobs all go crazy because of their problems?
- How does worrying help you to solve problems or prevent bad things happening?
- Is there any way to cope with problems without worrying?

Mindfulness, relaxation and exercise

Relaxation, meditation and regular physical exercise can all be helpful for managing GAD. Mindfulness allows people to take a more detached or non-judgemental view of worry thoughts, rather than getting 'caught up' or 'carried away' by their worries.

Social anxiety

People with social anxiety are fearful of embarrassment or humiliation and worry that others think badly of them or are judging them negatively. Situations that cause anxiety include talking to strangers or groups, doing things in front of people such as eating or performing, and going to meetings, classes, shops or social gatherings. Whilst some degree of anxiety before an important interview or a first date is normal, the anxiety experienced in social anxiety disorder is more severe and pervasive and it can be a highly disabling condition which undermines people's ability to interact with others.

Case Example 14.6: Social anxiety

Annette suffers from social anxiety in shops, restaurants and pubs. She hates waiting in a queue in the supermarket because she feels that everyone is watching her. She knows that it's not really true, but she can't shake the feeling, and she's terrified of doing something stupid and making a fool of herself. As she approaches the girl at the till, she tries to smile but her mouth is dry and her voice cracks. Annette is certain that the other shoppers must be staring and thinking how foolish she appears. Her hands shake and she drops her purse. Money rolls all over the floor. Her self-consciousness and anxiety rise to the roof. She decides never to return to the supermarket again.

Typical features of social anxiety

Thoughts

Patients with social anxiety worry about what others think of them and are fearful of saying or doing something 'wrong' in public. Socially anxious people hold negative beliefs about their ability in social situations. They tend to negatively misinterpret the thoughts and actions of others ('mind-reading') and assume that everyone is paying close attention to them and critically scrutinising what they are doing and saying. They tend to focus on their inner experiences and are highly self-conscious.

"I have nothing interesting to say. I'm boring."

"I'm shaking. Everyone is staring. They can all see I'm anxious."

"I will stammer/blush/go completely blank. I will look really stupid."

Feelings

Anxiety in social situations is associated with distressing feelings of embarrassment and shame.

Physical symptoms

Patients with social anxiety usually experience a range of physical symptoms such as blushing, sweating, shaking, rapid heartbeat, dry mouth and feeling light-headed or dizzy. These reactions make it difficult to concentrate and engage in social interaction and increase self-consciousness and worsen anxiety as a vicious cycle.

Behaviour

Typical behaviour includes avoidance or escape from anxiety-provoking situations and safety behaviours such as only talking to 'safe' people, trying to stay in the background, avoiding eye contact, speaking very quickly or never speaking in public. These behaviours restrict day to day activities, reduce confidence in their ability to cope in social situations and prevent the patient from learning that their negative thoughts and predictions were not really accurate.

CBT approaches to social anxiety

Focusing attention outwards

Socially anxious people spend a lot of time focusing on their inner reactions and bodily sensations to try to judge how anxious they may appear to others. This tends to worsen anxiety and also prevents the individual from fully engaging with the people and conversations around them.

Remind the patient that anxiety is often a lot less visible than they fear, and that others often have no idea how anxious they actually feel inside. It is more helpful to focus attention externally and concentrate on listening and engaging in the conversation rather than getting lost in their own thoughts and worries. *Box 14.6* contains some useful tips for managing social situations.

Changing unhelpful thinking patterns

Learning to identify and evaluate unhelpful thoughts can be a very important strategy in overcoming social anxiety (see *Box 14.7*).

The aim is to identify some alternative, balanced thoughts that help the person to face up to frightening situations (*Box 14.8*).

Reducing avoidance and safety behaviours

Changing behaviour is a key step in overcoming social anxiety. This involves gradually confronting social situations without relying on safety behaviours to cope. If the individual stays in the situation for long enough, their anxiety will

Box 14.6

Tips for managing social situations

- Try not to focus too much on what is going on inside you or how well you are performing. Instead, concentrate on listening and participating in the conversation that you are involved with.
- Remember that others may be far less aware of how anxious you feel. Anxiety is much less visible than you might think.
- Other people are not necessarily focusing on what you say or do. They are often far more self-focused and concerned with their own problems.
- Even if people notice you are anxious, it doesn't mean they will think badly of you. Everyone gets anxious sometimes. We don't have to perform 'perfectly' in every single conversation.
- Try to just be yourself and accept yourself 'warts and all'.

Box 14.7

Questions to help change unhelpful thinking in social anxiety

- What thoughts or fears arise during that situation? Are you jumping to the worst conclusion or 'catastrophising' in any way?
- Are you 'mind-reading' or assuming that you know what others are thinking? What evidence do you have that they think this? Is there any evidence to the contrary?
- Is there an alternative way to view the situation? What would a close friend say to you?
- What can you do next? What personal skills or strengths do you have that might help?

Box 14.8

Alternatives to negative thoughts

Negative thought	Balanced alternative
"I can't get my words out when I'm anxious. I sounded really stupid just then."	Everyone gets nervous sometimes. I did manage to say what I wanted to. Hesitating a bit doesn't make me stupid.
"My face went bright red. Everyone could see!"	People won't think less of me for blushing. They might not even have noticed – they may have been worrying about their own problems.

eventually reduce and this will boost their confidence to try new situations in future. Each time they face the situation it will become easier.

Encourage the patient to work upwards through a hierarchy of feared situations. They should try to remain in the situation until the anxiety reduces by at least half. This may take 30–45 minutes, although it often happens much more quickly. Each step should be repeated until it no longer causes significant anxiety. Then they move up to the next rung of the ladder.

Developing a compassionate inner voice

It may also be helpful for patients to work on developing a more compassionate inner voice that is less negative and self-critical and helps to improve their self-esteem and self-confidence (see *Chapter 18*).

Obsessive compulsive disorder

Obsessive compulsive disorder (OCD) involves recurrent thoughts (obsessions) and compulsive behaviours. An obsession is an unwanted, unpleasant thought, image or urge that repeatedly enters a person's mind, causing anxiety. These thoughts are interpreted by the patient as indicating that something bad might happen and that the individual is responsible for preventing it. Common thoughts in OCD relate to:

- worries about missing something potentially dangerous, such as forgetting to turn off the cooker or lock the front door
- fears of contamination, such as from touching a dirty surface or object
- excessive concern with order and perfection
- fear of uncontrollable or inappropriate behaviour in public, such as swearing or being violent.

To manage the anxiety that arises from these beliefs, the patient engages in compulsive safety behaviours, including avoidance and reassurance-seeking. OCD sufferers typically carry out various rituals involving cleaning, checking or repeating actions, and mental rituals such as thinking certain 'safe' thoughts. For example, someone with obsessive thoughts about catching a disease may compulsively wash their hands hundreds of times a day. These behaviours prevent the patient from learning that their fears are not really accurate.

In OCD, patients tend to assume excessive responsibility for preventing bad things from happening. They also overestimate the risk of a particular threat and find it difficult to tolerate uncertainty. 'Thought–action fusion' involves the belief that simply thinking about an action is equivalent to actually carrying it out, or that thinking about an unwanted event makes it more likely that the event will happen. For example, imagining a loved one dying in a car crash somehow makes it more likely that this will actually happen. Thought–action fusion makes it very difficult for patients with OCD to tolerate worrying thoughts.

> **Case Example 14.7: Obsessive compulsive disorder**
>
> Sian can remember worrying about germs, her health and the safety of others since childhood. She is very intelligent but is falling behind in her university course because she is constantly late or missing her classes altogether. She gets up at 6 am and spends the next 3 hours taking a long shower followed by repeatedly changing clothes until they 'feel right'. She packs and repacks her books over and over again and finally opens the front door. She then goes through a ritual of locking the door behind her and walking down the step, then walking back up again with a pause on each step and checking the lock once more. If she doesn't complete these rituals, she feels convinced that someone might break into the house and cause major harm to her family. Even though Sian recognises that her thoughts and behaviours are 'silly', she feels compelled to complete her rituals anyway. Finally, when finished, she has to rush to get to university and arrives halfway through the morning.

CBT interventions for OCD

OCD is typically a complex condition that is likely to require referral for specialist CBT services. CBT interventions that are beneficial in OCD include the following.

Exposure and response prevention

This involves 'exposure' of the patient to an object or situation that causes anxiety (e.g. touching a 'contaminated' object) whilst resisting carrying out the ritualistic behaviour (e.g. hand-washing). Over time, the exposure will lead to less and less anxiety ('habituation') and the patient learns that their feared outcome will not happen even if they do not carry out the safety behaviour.

Changing unhelpful thoughts, beliefs and behaviours

A thought record can be used to identify and evaluate obsessional thoughts (e.g. "*If I shake hands with someone, it will pass on germs and I will become seriously ill*"), and then coming up with a balanced new thought (e.g. "*Shaking hands is a safe activity and I am unlikely to get ill as a result*").

Challenging unhelpful beliefs about compulsive behaviour such as hand-washing can be carried out alongside behavioural experiments to test out the impact of changing these behaviours.

Key learning points

Summary of the cognitive behavioural model for anxiety:

Thoughts	Feelings
Fears of potential future danger	Anxiety and worry
Catastrophic and *'What if...?'* thoughts predicting the worst case scenario	Irritability, anger, frustration, guilt
	Low mood and depression
Underestimating own ability to cope with difficulties	
"I will have a heart attack or a stroke"	
"I will make a fool of myself or go mad"	
"Other people will think I am weak or stupid"	
Behaviour	**Physical symptoms**
Avoiding anxiety-provoking situations and people	Rapid heartbeat, palpitations
Safety behaviours (e.g. resting, staying with 'safe people')	Hyperventilation, feeling short of breath
Compulsive behaviour (e.g. checking, cleaning)	Chest pain, dry mouth, tightness in throat
	GI symptoms, feeling faint or dizzy; numbness and tingling, shaking
	Difficulty concentrating; feelings of unreality
Environment and background	
Stressful life events may trigger anxiety and panic attacks.	

- One of the most important messages for managing anxiety in primary care is to give credible, alternative explanations for anxiety-provoking symptoms such as a racing heart or chest pain.
- Emphasise that fear is a normal part of the 'fight or flight' response, which is designed to help us survive in the face of real physical danger. When the danger has passed, the anxiety will slowly fade away.
- Ensure that you tailor your explanations of anxiety to the patient's individual thoughts and physical experiences when anxious.

- Look for vicious cycles of negative thinking and unhelpful behaviour such as avoidance, escape or safety behaviours. Ask the patient how they might break this cycle.
- Facing anxiety-provoking situations in gradual stages helps the patient develop confidence to tackle more challenging situations. It is normal to feel some anxiety when trying these experiments and it is helpful to plan in advance how to cope with this, such as using controlled breathing or distraction. Over time the anxiety will reduce.
- Other useful strategies for managing anxiety include distraction, reducing reassurance and focusing on coping strategies rather than fears (e.g. constructing a *'then what...'* plan).

Chapter 15

Health anxiety and medically unexplained symptoms

Introduction

Medically unexplained symptoms

Medically unexplained symptoms (MUS) are physical symptoms that have no currently known pathological cause. These symptoms can be extremely debilitating and cause significant distress. Clinical presentations vary widely from people who regularly present with minor symptoms to people with severe disability, using wheelchairs or even becoming bed-bound.

Around 30% of patients with MUS have associated depression and anxiety. Patients with MUS may also have co-existing long-term physical health conditions. MUS can be categorised into three types, although there is much overlap.

- Health anxiety or hypochondriasis: a persistent fear of developing serious illness. Patients are highly anxious and remain convinced that they have a serious illness despite negative physical examinations, investigations and medical reassurance.
- Functional somatic disorders such as chronic back or pelvic pain, atypical chest pain, irritable bowel syndrome, chronic fatigue syndrome and fibromyalgia (see *Chapter 17*).
- Somatic symptoms presenting in patients with underlying anxiety or depression.

It is generally helpful to avoid using the term "MUS" with patients, as it may be seen as implying that the symptoms are not "real". Other potential terms include persistent physical symptoms and specific functional somatic syndromes, such as irritable bowel or chronic fatigue syndrome. If uncertain or lacking a diagnostic label, you can use descriptive terms such as "chronic facial pain" or "distressing sensation of dizziness".

Health anxiety and MUS in primary care

Physical symptoms with no known organic cause are common. In fact, most people have some daily physical sensations or symptoms, and 14–20% of primary care consultations involve a physical symptom without likely organic disease (Mumford *et al.*, 1991; Peveler *et al.*, 1997). However, the majority of these patients will not develop ongoing anxiety or persistent symptoms if managed appropriately by health professionals in the early stages of their presentation.

Smaller numbers of patients develop more persistent or severe problems. The prevalence of health anxiety is around 1–2% in the general population and 5–9% amongst GP attendees. This group may be responsible for disproportionately high usage of health services and can become a source of frustration, stress and 'heartsink' for health professionals (see *Chapter 19*).

Typical features of patients presenting with health anxiety and MUS in primary care are shown in *Box 15.1*:

Box 15.1	**Typical features of patients with health anxiety and MUS in primary care**

- Frequent attendances at GP surgeries, often associated with requests for repeated investigations and referrals.
- Multiple physical symptoms affecting functioning with no obvious cause.
- Vague, changing, unusual or atypical symptoms.
- Poor or variable response to multiple previous treatments.
- Past history is complex and difficult to clarify.

CBT for health anxiety and MUS

CBT is an effective treatment for health anxiety and MUS (Barsky & Ahern, 2004; Kroenke, 2007), which improves medical symptoms and associated symptoms of depression and anxiety. Nevertheless, there can be difficulties in offering talking treatments to patients who may not perceive their condition as being psychological in nature and are often fixed on seeking a medical cure for their problems.

A CBT approach to understanding health anxiety

Background/environmental factors

Individuals who lack social support, or were exposed to family conflict, illness or death during childhood are particularly vulnerable to developing health anxiety. Other associated factors include:

- maternal overprotection
- past experiences of unsatisfactory medical treatment
- lack of parental care or affection except when unwell
- severe cases can overlap with personality disorder (Bass & Murphy, 1995).

Illness behaviour may also be maintained by an element of 'secondary gain', including financial benefits, equipment, accommodation, and support or attention from friends, family and the medical profession.

Development of unhelpful core beliefs and rules about health

Health anxiety develops in vulnerable individuals when a *critical incident* activates underlying negative beliefs about health developed from past experiences. These beliefs include:

- viewing themselves as particularly vulnerable to illness (*"my body is weak and I am liable to develop something serious"*)
- fears about the experience of illness or death (*"I would not be able to cope with the agonising pain that always occurs in cancer"*)
- loss of self-esteem associated with a reduced ability to function normally through ill health (*"if I can't work through illness then I am a failure"*).

The development of health anxiety is shown in *Figure 15.1*.

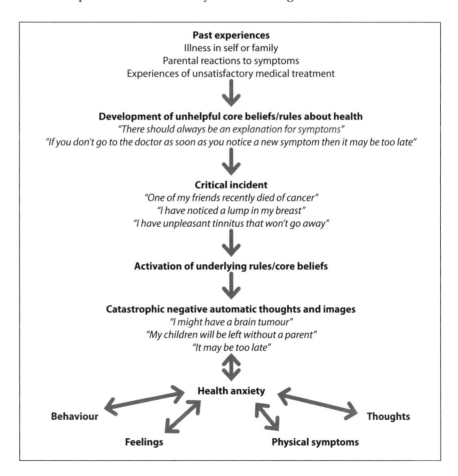

Figure 15.1: Development of health anxiety (Warwick & Salkovkis, 1989; Wells, 1997)

Case Example 15.1: The development of health anxiety

Denise is a social worker, who is married with three children. In February, she develops a flu-like illness lasting over a fortnight, where she feels feverish, weak and tired with aching muscles.

Background and predisposing factors

Denise was a premature baby who had several chest infections and was admitted to hospital at the age of 3 months. When she grew older, despite being in good health, her mother would keep her off school for minor illnesses, saying *"Your immune system is weak. We need to take special care of you."* Denise's mother would take her to the GP with any minor signs of illness. When Denise was 10 years old, her grandmother died unexpectedly. Her family was shocked and angry about her care in hospital.

In later life, Denise continued to worry about any minor symptom. Then her son developed a severe chest infection which required an overnight stay in hospital. Denise found this terrifying and it re-awakened many of her childhood fears about illness. Although her son recovered completely, Denise found it difficult to manage her own anxiety afterwards. Denise's own flu-like illness then acted as a trigger for the development of health anxiety.

Development of health anxiety

Denise only expected to be ill for a few days, so she was surprised that the illness lasted so long. A few weeks later she felt better, but not all the symptoms had gone. She felt weaker and became tired more quickly. She sometimes felt dizzy and noticed tingling in her hands and feet.

Denise visited her GP again, who tried to reassure her that there was nothing wrong, but her symptoms seemed to be getting worse. She found a magazine article about a woman with strange symptoms which turned out to be due to a brain tumour and she worried that the same might happen to her.

Denise imagined herself developing a severe illness such as multiple sclerosis. She had a frightening image of herself in a wheelchair, dependent on others and unable to care for her children. Whenever she had a quiet moment, Denise found herself thinking about becoming ill.

Denise returned to her GP several times and was referred to a neurologist. All the investigations were normal. Each time that Denise was reassured by a doctor or had a negative test, she felt hugely relieved. But she also felt compelled to keep checking and became anxious again if she noticed any symptoms (*"Tests and doctors can be wrong!"*).

> Denise spent a lot of time looking on the internet for medical information, and discovered a list of terrifying diseases that might be the cause of her symptoms. She visited many doctors who gave conflicting advice and often seemed uninterested in her problems.
>
> Because Denise felt so tired, she needed to rest a lot more. She kept checking her legs by tensing and relaxing the muscles, which made them achy and sore. *"My muscles are growing weaker"*, she thought, *"I'm getting worse"*. She stopped walking to work and avoided socialising with colleagues. At home she tended to sit down and spent less time playing with her children. She kept thinking *"If I feel this tired now, I will end up in a wheelchair in the future. My life will be ruined"*. This made her feel even more anxious and depressed.

Thoughts in health anxiety

Health anxious patients typically show a number of cognitive misperceptions, including:

- beliefs that particular illnesses are more likely or more serious than they are in reality (*"it might be cancer..."*)
- misinterpretation of harmless bodily symptoms as evidence of serious disease (*"the tiredness must be due to multiple sclerosis"*)
- viewing themselves as unable to prevent or cope with the illness if it did develop (*"I would be in excruciating, unbearable pain"*)
- constant thinking, worrying or talking about health maintains the focus on bodily symptoms, increasing anxiety and low mood
- focusing on information that confirms their fears whilst ignoring evidence of good health; this is a common cause of misunderstandings in medical communications (*"the doctor said it could be something serious"*).

Feelings and emotions

Patients with health anxiety experience high levels of anxiety about potential illness and its impact on their lives. They may also feel low or depressed. Feelings of anger and frustration are also common, and may be directed towards health professionals, who are perceived as ignoring a genuine, severe medical problem.

Physical symptoms and reactions

Any physical symptom can be associated with anxiety, depending on what meaning a patient assigns to it. Patients misinterpret normal variations in bodily sensations, or symptoms related to a benign condition such as tinnitus, as a sign of serious ill health. They also experience anxiety-related physical symptoms, which are also misinterpreted as evidence of physical illness. Fatigue and muscle aches can arise due to reduced activity and loss of fitness. Side-effects of medication can also lead to unpleasant physical sensations.

The role of behaviour

Behaviour in health anxiety is generally designed to check for or protect from physical illness. However, these reactions just maintain or worsen the patient's anxiety. Common behaviour in health anxiety includes the following.

- *Reassurance-seeking*: seeking constant reassurance from health professionals, family and friends can temporarily reduce anxiety, but leads to a longer-term increase in fear and the need for further reassurance as a vicious cycle.
- *Body-checking and scanning*: patients constantly monitor and check their body for 'danger' symptoms and signs of disease. This often causes new symptoms such as pain, redness or swelling. Patients also notice normal variations in bodily functions, and interpret all these sensations as evidence of serious ill-health.
- *Frequent attendance at health services*: patients make frequent visits to multiple health professionals, requesting repeated investigations and referrals. These may temporarily reassure the patient, but ultimately *increase* anxiety (*"the doctor must think it's serious or they wouldn't do a test"*) and reinforce beliefs about the need for medical tests to investigate symptoms. It can also cause frustration on both sides and prevent the patient from building a trusting relationship with one health professional.
- *Behaving 'as if' they are ill*: illness behaviours such as reducing activity, using inappropriate medication, using a wheelchair or taking an illness role in family life, reinforce the patient's belief that they really are unwell. The associated reduction in enjoyable and meaningful activities also worsens any tiredness and low mood.
- *Thinking, talking and reading about health*: patients may spend a great deal of time reading medical information in books, magazines and on the internet. This worsens anxiety as they become aware of other potentially serious medical problems. Talking excessively about health problems also maintains their preoccupation with illness.
- *Avoidance*: some anxious individuals try to avoid reminders of physical illness to suppress their fears. However, attempts at thought suppression or avoidance are usually unsuccessful and often result in a paradoxical increase in unwanted thoughts, which seem more frightening than ever.

From *theory* to *practice*...

- Think about a patient that you regularly see who is often anxious about their health. Then try to build a simple 'case formulation' by mapping out their difficulties using the five areas of the CBM.
- What typical thoughts, feelings and behaviours are associated with the person's physical symptoms?
- Which environmental factors, both past and present, might be relevant to the development of the disorder in this individual?
- Is the patient trapped in any vicious cycles?
- Finish by identifying one simple next step that you might take for trying to understand this patient and build a rapport with them.

Managing MUS and health anxiety

Steps for a CBT approach to MUS

1. Build a trusting relationship with the patient.
2. Review and summarise the patient's medical notes.
3. Conduct a longer status consultation in which you:
   - begin by reviewing physical symptoms
   - explore thoughts, feelings, physical symptoms, behaviour, environmental factors and triggers
   - include summarising, link-making and handover questions.
4. Give empowering explanations for all symptoms.
5. Broaden the agenda.
6. Negotiate treatment (medical and non-medical).
7. Ask for feedback / check patient understanding at the end of the consultation.
8. Use appropriate CBT-based strategies (e.g. goal setting).

Build a trusting relationship with patients

One of the most important goals for health professionals is to build rapport and a trusting relationship with patients with MUS. Focus on being empathic, warm, concerned and respectful, using non-judgemental language and trying to work in partnership with the patient to overcome their difficulties. Take time to learn about the person's life, family, pets and interests. *Box 15.2* highlights some common pitfalls to avoid for health professionals working with MUS patients.

Set realistic goals

It is important to set realistic goals for working with patients with MUS and health anxiety. Focus on making small steps forwards. For many patients, a

Box 15.2

What not to do – medical behaviour that worsens health anxiety

- Not giving a credible explanation for the patient's symptoms or using only negative statements (*"there is nothing wrong with you"*).
- Behaviour suggesting that you do not believe the patient or take their symptoms seriously.
- Blaming the patient for their problems.
- Giving excessive reassurance which does not address the fears underlying the individual patient's anxiety.
- Carrying out repeated unnecessary investigations or referrals to specialists.
- Giving unnecessary strong or addictive medication.

highly appropriate goal is to stabilise their condition and prevent further deterioration or iatrogenic harm.

Ensure the primary care team works together as a whole

Encourage patients to see one lead health professional on a regular basis who can get to know them well. These clinicians may require team support through practice meetings and discussions. Try to proactively arrange appointments in advance rather than allowing the patient to book on an *ad hoc* basis.

It is also essential to communicate clearly with all members of the team and specialists. Write clear notes about agreed management plans and give the patient clear, written instructions on who to contact and how to manage flare-ups or likely changes in symptoms.

Case Example 15.2: Introducing a 10 Minute CBT approach to health anxiety

Victoria is a 26 year old teacher whose father died from lung cancer when she was a child. She has become increasingly anxious about her own health since a family friend was recently diagnosed with breast cancer. Victoria is worried about her recurrent headaches, despite having been diagnosed with tension-type headaches by a neurologist. She attends the GP surgery regularly, asking for further tests to check that her symptoms are not serious.

Victoria Hello Doctor. I need you to do something about my headaches!

GP How were you hoping that I might help you today?

Victoria These headaches must be something serious. I'd like to have some more tests to check them out.

GP	I've noticed that you have come in several times recently about your headaches, even though you got the 'all clear' from the specialist.
Victoria	He might have made a mistake. It's not normal to get headaches so often.
GP	You seem really worried.
Victoria	I am worried. You read about this all the time – doctors missing things that turn out to be serious.
GP	We have spent quite a bit of time looking into the cause of your headaches, but that doesn't seem to be helping you to feel any better.
Victoria	Well, I can't stop thinking that they might mean something really bad.
GP	I wonder if, as well as continuing to treat your headaches, we should spend some time trying to help you feel less anxious when you have one. This doesn't mean that we stop giving you the medical care that you need. But, it might also be helpful to spend some time understanding why they are causing you so much worry, despite all the negative tests.
Victoria	Tests can be wrong! I would feel better if I could be sure that there is nothing bad causing them, or get rid of them altogether.
GP	It is very common to get headaches, so it may not be possible to get rid of them altogether. And feeling anxious and stressed about having them might actually make them worse.
Victoria	I suppose that's true. But mine are really bad.
GP	They sound very distressing. Would you be prepared to make an appointment in 2 weeks, to fully review your headaches and how they are affecting your life?
Victoria	Yes, I would be glad to come and talk about this. It's really starting to get me down.

Review and summarise the patient's notes

Before you see the patient it can be helpful to read and summarise the patient's prior history, investigations and treatments including:

- previous disease episodes and clusters of symptoms
- hospital letters and discharge summaries
- tests and results
- mental health problems and psychosocial triggers
- patterns of disease and symptom severity over time in relation to external stress and events in the patient's life.

This summary should be highlighted in the medical records for anyone who might see the patient. Although it may seem like a time-consuming exercise, this information can save a huge amount of time and enable far better clinical decision-making.

Carry out a longer 'status consultation'

The next step is to arrange a longer 20–30 minute initial consultation with a patient with MUS. Start with a thorough review of the patient's physical symptoms and carry out a physical examination if needed. Use this session as a 'fact-finding mission' and try to avoid offering diagnoses, opinions or suggestions at this stage. Make a written list of key symptoms and ask about a typical day or for specific examples of when symptoms were particularly troublesome. Don't rush this step. It may take the entire first consultation to review the physical symptoms.

The aim is to build a relationship and ensure the patient feels understood and listened to, using empathic and reflective statements to acknowledge the reality and distressing nature of the symptoms. The next step is to explore all five areas of the cognitive behavioural model (see *Figure 15.2* which includes some useful questions).

Thoughts	Feelings
"What went through your mind when you noticed the symptoms?" *"What is your biggest concern or fear that these symptoms might mean?"* *"What troubles you most about your symptoms?"*	*"How does it make you feel to have these symptoms?"* *"How do you feel when you think, 'It might be cancer'?"* *"These symptoms seem to be causing you a great deal of worry..."* Include empathic statements: *"That must be very difficult..."*
Behaviour	**Physical symptoms**
"What do you do when you notice the symptoms?" *"What do you do to make yourself feel better?"* *"Do you test or check your health in any way?"* *"Do you talk to others or read up about your health?"* *"What are you doing differently now? Is there anything you are no longer doing?"*	*"Tell me about the physical symptoms that trouble you the most"* *"Are there any other important symptoms?"*
Background, environment and triggers	
"Is there anything else going on in your life that is making the symptoms difficult to cope with?" *"Was anything going on at the time that they first started?"* *"Has anything happened in your life to make you particularly concerned about your health?"*	

Figure 15.2: Questions to explore the five areas of the CBM in health anxiety

Some patients with MUS have difficulty in discussing emotional factors, and may hold unhelpful beliefs about expressing emotions. In this case, do not overemphasise emotional aspects of the problem, and instead focus on discussing physical and behavioural issues.

Finish by summarising what you have heard and checking that the patient understands and agrees with you. Gently highlight any links or vicious cycles (see *Figure 15.3*) that you have noticed:

> *"You mentioned that when you think 'It might be cancer,' you start to feel quite anxious."*

Always follow a summary with a handover question which encourages the patient to reflect on the discussion.

> *"What do you make of this? Is there any way we can use this information to help you?"*

Provide empowering explanations for key symptoms

Giving clear, concrete and tangible explanations of symptoms can help to reduce health anxiety. Avoid jargon and link your explanation to any specific fears or health beliefs held by a particular patient. If there is no easy medical explanation, then give clear reasons why the symptoms do not fit with something serious.

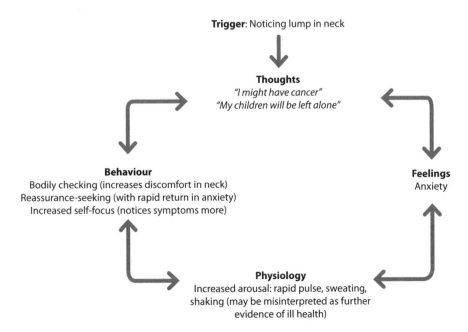

Figure 15.3: Example of a vicious cycle in a patient with health anxiety

It is helpful to provide written information, but simply handing the patient a leaflet does not constitute an empowering explanation! Try to provide the information in the form of a dialogue, checking understanding as you proceed.

Explicitly acknowledge that the patient's symptoms are real and a source of major concern and distress. However, you can also emphasise that the severity of symptoms is not necessarily an indicator of the seriousness of the underlying condition.

> *"I know that you are worried that your pain is due to a problem with your heart, but I believe that it is coming from the muscles in your chest wall. When these muscles go into spasm it can be extremely painful. However, having severe pain does not necessarily mean a serious or dangerous underlying cause."*

If possible, include options for self-help or self-management of the symptoms (*Box 15.3*).

Box 15.3

Empowering explanations of symptoms

- Physical tension or anxiety can lead to pain.
- Stress at home causes tension in the muscles of your back and this can lead to pain.
- Depression lowers the pain threshold and makes pain worse (see *Chapter 12*).
- When you feel low or depressed your body becomes more sensitive to pain so it feels more intense. Could that be true for you?
- Thinking about symptoms makes them worse.
- Constantly thinking about or touching the affected area makes it feel even worse.

Coping with uncertainty

Health anxious patients often say that they would like to be 100% *certain* that nothing serious is wrong. However, it is impossible to completely eliminate the risk of developing any disease, no matter how rare it may be. Constantly thinking about the worst case scenario does not reduce the risk of it occurring and life becomes filled with anxiety and stress. Instead, emphasise living in the 'here and now'.

> *"I understand that the idea of having a heart problem makes you feel very anxious and that you would like to feel certain that your heart is 100% healthy. All the tests do confirm that. However, we all live with some uncertainty about health because we can never guarantee that we will not*

become ill in the future. Worry will not prevent this. It is important that the fear of becoming ill does not prevent you from living a fulfilling and enjoyable life. How much time do you spend worrying about developing an illness? Do you think this is helping you? Suppose you spend the next 10 years worrying about getting cancer but do not develop it? Would this worry have been a good use of your time?"

Rather than continually reassuring the patient, try to share the uncertainty with them. People are often more willing to accept uncertainty about a diagnosis if you provide assurance that you will keep an open mind and their symptoms will be taken seriously and reassessed in future if things change.

"I take your health very seriously and I will be happy to review this again if needed."

Broaden the agenda

The next stage is to broaden the patient's perspective to incorporate the idea that their problem is not purely an undiagnosed physical health condition, but also includes caring for emotional wellbeing and finding ways to live a fulfilling and meaningful life despite the presence or absence of physical symptoms.

Avoid black and white perspectives of the problem being *either* medical *or* psychological in nature. Instead, reassure the patient that you will continue to treat physical health problems with a holistic approach which includes medical treatment as well as additional strategies which may help them to cope more effectively with their symptoms.

"It also strikes me that the worry and stress about your symptoms is causing as much problem as the symptoms themselves, what do you think...?"

"You've been suffering from this for a long time. Doing tests and referrals doesn't seem to be helping you to feel better. Perhaps we could try a different approach...?"

"It seems that the symptoms are having a major impact on your life. Perhaps we could look at some ways of helping to improve the quality of your life, even if the symptoms are still present..."

Avoid falling into the trap of continually debating the cause of symptoms, or trying to convince the patient that their problems are *really* psychological in nature. Instead, try to explore and acknowledge the patient's fears about the meaning of symptoms.

"I see that you are worrying about your symptoms again. What thoughts are going through your mind? That must be very distressing."

Negotiate the next steps (medical and non-medical treatments)

Primary care management of health anxious patients is likely to involve a variety of approaches including medication, investigations, referrals and psychological strategies. Involve the patient in decision-making wherever possible. The main focus should be on managing symptoms and improving functioning. Remember also to proactively screen for and treat mental health disorders such as depression according to guidelines.

Primary care management involves investigating symptoms appropriately and thoroughly but without excessive repetition of tests or referrals simply 'for reassurance'. Telling a patient beforehand that you are expecting a normal result may help them to feel more reassured by a negative test. Try to minimise the use of medication, particularly if it is potentially addictive or has serious side-effects. Relevant information to include in a referral letter is shown in *Box 15.4*.

Positive risk management involves balancing the risk of over-investigation with that of missed diagnoses. Avoid making assumptions and use your clinical judgement to assess and manage any new or changing symptoms. Inform and document clearly about 'red flag' symptoms and signs.

Box 15.4	**Key information to include in referral letters for patients with MUS**
	• Inform the specialist that you suspect possible MUS.
	• Be clear what you are asking them (e.g. to rule out a specific illness).
	• Include details of relevant psychosocial factors.
	• Provide a detailed past medical history including MUS syndromes and mental health problems.

Check patient understanding

Always finish by checking what the patient has understood from the consultation. Remember, she may believe that you said she has a serious physical illness. Try to respond without being defensive.

> *"I'm glad you were able to share that with me because that wasn't the impression I was hoping to give you. In fact, I don't think it is likely that your symptoms are due to cancer. I believe that they are due to an unpleasant but harmless condition called irritable bowel syndrome..."*

CBT strategies for managing MUS

The main aims for managing MUS in primary care should be to improve function and quality of life, even if symptoms are persistent and remain unexplained.

Behavioural strategies in health anxiety

Promoting behavioural change is possibly the most important and realistic strategy for dealing with health anxiety in primary care. This includes changing unhelpful patterns of behaviour and setting goals to increase meaningful and enjoyable activities despite the presence of symptoms.

Graded exercise and relaxation

A graded stretching and exercise programme can be extremely effective at improving fitness and reducing symptoms such as fatigue and muscle pain. This should follow principles of paced activity to avoid 'boom and bust' patterns of behaviour. Try to encourage the patient to draw on social support to maintain exercise over time; for example, walking with friends or a local group. This will help to motivate them to keep up the changes and the increased social interaction may also help to lift their mood.

Relaxation and mindfulness may also be very helpful for improving symptom control.

Goal setting

It is important for patients to gradually resume their normal daily activities. This is likely to boost mood, increase the level of enjoyment in life, give an increased sense of satisfaction and take their minds off negative thoughts and worries.

The next step is to jointly plan some goals for improving life, even if symptoms remain. Goals should relate to the patient's values and important life areas (see *Chapter 8*). Ask the patient:

> "What was life like before you developed these symptoms? What did you used to enjoy?"

> "What matters most in your life? What activities might be important for you to build up again...?"

> "What would you do differently if you felt better?"

> "Could you try any of these in very small steps...?"

It can be helpful to monitor current activity levels and plan future changes using a behaviour monitoring chart (see *Chapter 7*).

Reducing reassurance-seeking behaviour

Health professionals should try to avoid getting drawn into constant demands for reassurance from health anxious patients. It is often more helpful to reflect back what they say with an empathic statement:

Patient *I just need to be sure it is not cancer*
GP *It sounds like you are worrying about cancer again. That must be very difficult.*

Reducing reassurance-seeking behaviour should be planned collaboratively with the patient, and involve both family members and health professionals. Instead of asking for reassurance, the patient could try an alternative activity or distraction exercise. They could also try reviewing some pre-written information, such as a thought record, reassuring statements, pie chart or written strategies for how to cope with anxiety-provoking situations.

Reducing monitoring and body-checking

Ask patients to record in a journal how often they check a particular aspect of their physical health each day. The next step is to agree how much body-checking is *helpful* for the future. For example, if the patient fears cancer, then checking once a month is more appropriate than several times an hour.

It is often difficult to stop body-checking, which may have become an ingrained habit. Techniques such as distraction or using thought records to find alternatives for negative thoughts can be useful. Patients can also remind themselves that body checking is increasing their anxiety in the long term.

From *theory* to *practice*...

Investigating the effect of reassurance
Ask patients with health anxiety to observe the effects of other people's reassurance on their anxiety. Does reassurance reduce their anxiety? How long does this last for?

Does being reassured reduce any of their physical symptoms? How can they explain this? Would a serious diagnosis be likely to go away simply with reassurance?

Is there any way that you could *permanently* reassure them? Why not? What does this tell them about the nature of their worry?

Monitoring and body-checking behaviour
Ask patients to notice what happens when they focus internally on symptoms or their body state. How does this alter their thoughts or anxiety levels? What is the impact of continually poking and prodding the skin or of continually taking forced, deep breaths? How might this contribute to their anxiety problems?

Cognitive strategies for health anxiety

Using a pie chart to generate alternative ideas for symptoms

A pie chart can be a powerful visual tool which encourages the patient to keep in mind the most common and likely causes of particular symptoms. Use guided discovery to encourage patients to think up a range of possible causes and to draw their own conclusions from the exercise.

Case Example 15.2: *Continued*: using pie charts to look for alternative explanations for symptoms

Let's return to the example of Victoria, the young woman with headaches and health anxiety.

Her GP encourages her to generate a list of common causes for headaches:

- stress and tension
- migraine
- eye strain / bright light
- loud noise
- bang on the head
- blocked sinuses
- brain tumour

Next, Victoria's GP draws a large circle and asks Victoria to divide up the 'pie' into slices. Each slice represents how common the different causes are and how likely to have caused headaches in a woman of her age. She leaves her most feared cause (a brain tumour) until *last* to put on the chart. She draws the following pie chart:

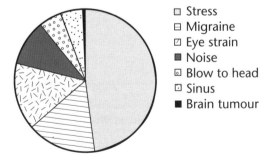

□ Stress
⊟ Migraine
▨ Eye strain
■ Noise
▣ Blow to head
▢ Sinus
■ Brain tumour

After this exercise, Victoria's GP asks her, 'What do you make of this chart?' Victoria replies that it is helpful to think about all the possible causes of her illness rather than focusing on the one or two, most serious possibilities.

Note: the sections of the chart need only be approximate. However, if the patient is vastly overestimating the likelihood of one particular cause, it may be helpful to discuss this openly.

Looking for evidence for and against specific, feared diagnoses

Written thought records (*Box 15.5*) can be used to look for evidence for and against particular negative thoughts or feared diagnoses.

Box 15.5

Using thought records to test out unhelpful thoughts in health anxiety

Thought to test out
My headaches are due to a brain tumour.

Evidence *for* having a brain tumour	Evidence *against* having a brain tumour
The headaches I get are very severe.	Brain tumours are very rare – there are many other causes of headaches and most are not serious.
I have had them for a long time.	I have had lots of tests, including a brain scan. These were all normal.
Doctors do make mistakes and sometimes miss serious illnesses.	The headache gets better if I lie down and rest – brain tumours would not get better so easily.
	My headaches are worse when I am stressed or anxious – this does not fit with a brain tumour.
	The doctor says that I do not have any other signs that would indicate a brain tumour.

Alternative / balanced thought to replace the hot thought
My headaches are more likely to be due to tension and stress. Worrying about my headaches makes them worse and makes me feel very anxious.

Theory A and Theory B method

- Theory A: this is a worry I have about my symptoms and when I worry and pay attention to them they get worse.
- Theory B: the symptoms are dangerous and serious.

Discuss both theories openly with the patient. Look for evidence for both and write them down or talk through them to decide which theory best fits the facts.

Other methods of coping with health anxiety and worry

- Encourage acceptance of uncertainty about health, which enables people to face up to scary thoughts and make more positive choices and develop coping strategies.
- Use distraction to focus the mind on other things.
- Focus on coping strategies rather than fears. Use a 'then what..?' approach to identify ways to cope with feared outcomes. For example, discussing how to cope if they did develop a particular disorder.
- Use mindfulness to distance from scary thoughts, difficult emotions and unpleasant symptoms ('See your thoughts, don't be your thoughts').
- Plan a designated 'worry time' each day (as for generalised anxiety disorder, see *Chapter 14*).

Key learning points

Summary of the cognitive behavioural model for health anxiety:

Unhelpful core beliefs and rules about health	
"I am vulnerable to illness"	
"Being ill means that something serious is likely to happen"	
"If I can't do my job through ill-health then my life is ruined"	
Thoughts	**Feelings**
Serious illnesses are more likely than in reality	Anxiety and worry
Harmless symptoms viewed as evidence of ill-health	Irritability, anger, frustration
Belief that unable to prevent or cope with the illness	Low mood and depression
Constant thinking about health (preoccupation with health)	
Ignore evidence of good health	

Behaviour	Physical symptoms
Frequent visits to multiple health professionals	Physical symptoms associated with benign conditions
Reassurance-seeking and avoidance	Anxiety-related somatic symptoms
Excessive talking and reading about health	
Body-checking and scanning	Tiredness and fatigue due to reduced activity
Illness behaviours	Side-effects from medication

Environment and background
Maternal overprotection, lack of parental care or affection except when unwell; past experiences of unsatisfactory medical treatment
Critical incident activates health anxiety (e.g. unexpected illness in self or others)

- Health anxiety arises from a persistent fear of serious illness. Patients experience genuine physical symptoms but overestimate the likely severity of the cause.
- A patient with a health anxiety disorder will feel anxious despite negative physical examinations, tests or medical reassurance, so try not to feel frustrated, but view it as an understandable response based on a psychological model of the disorder.
- Work on developing effective and trusting relationships between GP and patient. Listen and acknowledge the reality and distressing nature of symptoms.
- Try not to contribute to the vicious cycle of worsening health anxiety with inappropriate investigations, unsatisfactory explanations or excessive reassurance. Consider psychological referral.
- Be realistic with your goals. It may be most appropriate to aim to prevent further deterioration or iatrogenic harm.
- The main focus for change should be to encourage improved function and wellbeing despite the presence of persistent symptoms. Encourage graded increase in meaningful and valued activities, particularly involving exercise and social interaction.

Chapter 16

Chronic physical disease

The psychological impact of chronic disease

Emotional disorders are common in patients with physical disease. Around 20–25% of patients with chronic medical problems experience clinically significant psychological symptoms such as depression or anxiety (Craig & Boardman, 1997). However, health professionals often focus predominantly on the physical rather than the emotional health of patients with chronic disease, and depression is more likely to be missed or overlooked in these patients.

Developing chronic illness or disability is likely to require major changes in people's attitudes and lives. Patients must learn to cope with their disease, its associated symptoms, and any impact on their usual daily functioning. They may need to make psychosocial adjustments in order to maintain independence and previous roles at work and in the family. Patients must also learn to understand and manage their condition. Some treatments produce unpleasant side-effects or require unwelcome life changes. People with chronic disease must also deal with uncertainty as to the possible future or prognosis of the illness.

The role of health beliefs in adjusting to chronic disease

People's beliefs about the diagnosis, symptoms, severity, duration and cause of their illness, as well as their views about the value or role of medical or other treatments, will affect how they make sense of their illness. These beliefs influence individual coping strategies, behavioural reactions to illness, compliance with treatment and the emotional impact of health problems.

Certain beliefs about illness may predispose the patient to becoming depressed, anxious or angry in the face of real or potential illness, for example:

"Being unable to work through ill health means I have nothing to offer."

"Others think less of me for being ill."

"Medications are dangerous and should be avoided."

"Nothing can help me. Things are only going to get worse."

"I can only feel better if I am completely free from all symptoms."

These negative health beliefs result in unhelpful coping strategies and safety behaviours such as lack of compliance with treatment, excessive reassurance-seeking and social withdrawal. These behavioural patterns lead to worsening low mood, increased anxiety and low self-esteem.

Developing more adaptive health beliefs can reduce emotional distress in the face of physical illness, for example:

"I am a worthwhile, valuable person, despite changes in my life such as no longer working."

"Medications may sometimes be necessary to help my body."

"Others will still respect and care for me if I become unwell."

"The worst may not happen."

"I can cope with the problems that I am facing."

Using 10 minute CBT with physical illness and disability

The goal for managing chronic disease is to promote independence and enjoyable living, *despite* the presence of physical illness. This may involve learning to accept alterations in body function, appearance and lifestyle, without associating these changes with a loss of personal worth or value. An essential aspect of a CBT approach is to increase the patient's ability to understand and manage their own physical and emotional symptoms (improved self-management and self-efficacy).

Identifying and then changing unhelpful behaviour patterns is a key strategy for making change. For example, patients may behave 'as if' they are more unwell or disabled than is really the case, which limits activity and can worsen mood.

Acceptability of psychological approaches to physical disorders

Primary healthcare professionals are in an ideal position to offer emotional support to patients with physical health conditions, who may be unwilling to engage with psychological services. You can reassure the patient that discussing psychological or emotional aspects of problems will be combined with standard medical approaches and treatment of their condition.

"Alongside managing your physical health as usual, would it also be helpful to discuss how you are feeling about your illness and how to help you feel less anxious?"

"Many people find that physical symptoms become even worse if they feel low. Perhaps it would be helpful to discuss this...?"

Case Example 16.1: Using the CBM in diabetes

Donald is a 56 year old, overweight decorator who was diagnosed with type II diabetes last year during a routine health check. His blood sugar readings indicate that his diabetes is poorly controlled but he does not appear interested in his illness. Donald's GP suspects that he is not taking his medication regularly, because he rarely asks for a repeat prescription. But whenever the practice nurse tries to educate him about diabetes and encourage him to take his medication, he gets irritated and aggressive, saying that he has heard it all before.

Donald's GP decides to use a 10 minute CBT approach to understand Donald's reluctance to discuss diabetes or take his medication.

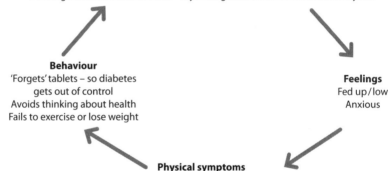

Thoughts
"Having diabetes means that I am 'ill' and my body is weak and out of control."
"If I think too much about diabetes it will take over my life – better to ignore it."
"It is dangerous to take medications – my uncle got an ulcer from his tablets last year."

Behaviour
'Forgets' tablets – so diabetes
gets out of control
Avoids thinking about health
Fails to exercise or lose weight

Feelings
Fed up / low
Anxious

Physical symptoms
Tired and lethargic

Environment
Donald doesn't really enjoy his job – *"It pays the bills"*
His friends are mainly in his local pub – most drink quite heavily
His wife is also overweight and tends to cook rich and fatty food

By understanding Donald better, his GP feels less frustrated and is able to express genuine empathy for the patient's difficulties. This helps improve their relationship, and encourages Donald to attend the diabetic clinic more regularly. Donald and his GP discuss the evidence for and against his beliefs about diabetes and develop some alternative, more helpful thoughts, such as, *"Taking medications could protect me from serious harm from diabetes"* and *"Ignoring problems doesn't make them go away."*

The GP also uses goal setting and motivational interviewing techniques to facilitate Donald in making lifestyle changes such as increasing exercise and weight loss (*see Chapter 8*).

Case Example 16.2: Low mood in multiple sclerosis

Diane is a 45 year old woman with multiple sclerosis. Her physical strength and mobility have gradually reduced over the past 5 years and she is now largely confined to a wheelchair. She is married with two children and feels increasingly low about her loss of independence and difficulty carrying out her normal tasks of daily living. She is no longer able to play physical games with her children, or to lift her younger son, Ivan, aged 4.

Thoughts	*"I'm a terrible mum – I can't even play with the children any more."* *"I've failed my family."* *"Things are only going to get worse in the future."*
Feelings	Guilt, depression
Behaviour	Reduced interaction with her children which reinforces her belief about being a 'bad' parent. Frequently mentions her perceived 'failure' to her husband, Barry. This makes him feel anxious and low, so he usually responds by changing the subject. Diane views this reaction as 'evidence' that he agrees with her negative self-view
Physical symptoms	Increasing tiredness and lethargy Muscular fatigue and weakness

Strategies that Diane's GP could use to help her feel less depressed include:

- behavioural activation and activity scheduling – increase positive and meaningful activities
- increase social interaction and encourage Diane to seek support from friends and family members
- use of thought records and diaries to identify and evaluate negative or unhelpful thoughts
- use positive diaries or lists of personal qualities to build self-esteem, despite the presence of illness.

Managing complex physical and emotional problems

Write a problem list

Patients with chronic disease often have a complex mix of physical and emotional problems, which can be confusing and overwhelming for both

GP and patient. Writing a problem list is a helpful way to make sense of complex problems. It can make difficulties seem more manageable and can help a patient to prioritise which areas to focus on first. Sometimes patients will realise that several problems on the list are related and that their list of difficulties is not as long as they feared.

The first step is to write a list of all the patient's problems. The patient can be asked to prioritise these problems and decide which ones to address first. The next step is to explore the key problems in greater depth. This should include an assessment of practical, physical, psychological and emotional aspects of problems. Ask the patient to reflect on what bothers them the most about their problems or physical symptoms (*Box 16.1*):

Box 16.1

Exploring problem areas in more depth

- *"What would you most like to change? If we could work together to improve something, what would this be?"*
- *"What makes this a problem for you? What bothers you the most about it?"*
- *"Can you give me a recent example? What happened…?"*
- *"How do you think/feel/react? How do others react?"*
- *"What makes it better/worse?"* (include cognitive/behavioural/ situational factors)
- *"Does it occur at particular times or in specific situations?"*
- *"Are there times that this is less of a problem for you? What are these?"*
- What particular beliefs does the patient hold about themselves, their illness, medical staff, etc., which might be associated with this problem?

Case Example 16.3: Using a problem list for a patient with chronic disease

Jean is a 58 year old accounts clerk. She is overweight and has hypertension. She has arthritis of the knees and is awaiting a knee replacement. Her knees are very painful and she sometimes takes non-steroidal anti-inflammatory medication, but has gastrointestinal side-effects. This limits how often she can take them.

Jean's problem list:
1. arthritis in knees
2. need to lose weight
3. husband had a heart attack last year
4. problems at work
5. feeling increasingly fed up and depressed

In the following dialogue, Jean and her GP discuss the impact of her worsening arthritis on her life.

GP	Which of these problems do you see as the most important to discuss first?

GP Which of these problems do you see as the most important to discuss first?

Jean Well, life has become very difficult now that the arthritis in my knees has got so bad.

GP In what ways has this become a problem for you?

Jean I just can't do as much as I used to.

GP And what kinds of physical symptoms stop you…?

Jean I'm in a lot of pain. I also feel so tired nowadays.

GP Can you tell me what kind of things you are no longer doing, since you developed the arthritis? What did you used to do differently?

Jean I used to be very active. I was always out and about seeing friends. Now I hardly get out at all and I don't see my friends very often these days.

GP How does it make you feel not to be able to do these things any more?

Jean It makes me feel really fed up and down. Sometimes I get very angry about it.

GP I see. Can you tell me what makes you feel fed up? What goes through your mind when you feel that way?

Jean I think that my life is over. I'm only 58 but my life is so empty and meaningless now.

GP I understand. It must be very difficult to cope with the pain. I'd like to briefly summarise what you told me about your problems so far:
You said that your arthritis is causing you a lot of pain and that you also feel very tired. Because of this, you are hardly able to get out and see your friends, which makes you feel very fed up and low, because you are thinking that "My life is over. I'm only 58 but my life is empty and meaningless."
What do you make of all this? Is there anything you might be able to do to make any changes in this…?

Jean I can see how I really miss getting out of the house and seeing my friends. But it's so difficult with my arthritis.

GP It seems like you have got rather stuck. I wonder if there is any way that you might be able to make your life seem more enjoyable and worthwhile, even if you still continue to have the arthritis and pain?

Jean I hadn't really thought about it like that before. But I can see that it would make me feel better if I had more enjoyable things in my life. I will have to think about what I could still do.

GP That sounds like a really good idea. Perhaps we could make a list of suggestions…

Jean and her GP repeated this discussion on several occasions, to construct the following table showing her most important problems.

Problem	Arthritis in knees	Need to lose weight	Husband had a heart attack last year
Physical symptoms associated	Pain, especially after walking Stiffness Tired and lethargic Poor sleep	Makes arthritis worse Easily tired	Tense Poor sleep
Thoughts about problem	"I'm in too much pain to enjoy life." "I can't do anything that I used to." "My life has really changed."	"Eating is my only pleasure in life these days." "I can't do any activity because of pain in my knees." "There's no point in trying – I will never manage to change anything."	"What if he has another one?" "I couldn't cope alone." "I am responsible for keeping him well." "He needs to constantly rest in order to protect his heart."
Feelings associated with problem	Frustrated Fed up / low	Guilty Low	Anxious Worried
Ways of behaving	Stopped walking to work Gradually cut down leisure activities Less social interaction	Try to 'be good' but frequent snacks Frequently gives up dieting Reduce activity, including enjoyable ones	Frightened to leave him alone: "what if he has another heart attack while I am out?" Does most housework – "my husband must be allowed to rest."

By gradually building up an understanding of her problems, Jean is able to identify some simple ways to try to overcome some of these difficulties, including:

- increasing time spent undertaking enjoyable activities or hobbies, despite the presence of pain
- gradually increasing gentle exercise such as swimming, which does not worsen knee pain
- focusing on a healthy eating plan, rather than extreme 'yo-yo' dieting regimes
- encouraging husband to take on more responsibility for jobs around the home ("*It is important to build up strength after a heart attack, rather than constantly resting*"). This may boost his self-esteem and gives Jean more time to focus on herself.

Coping with uncertainty

Coping with uncertainty is an inevitable part of living with nearly every physical disorder. Some patients can accept this uncertainty as inevitable. They may be able to 'live for the moment' by focusing on what they *do* know rather than constantly worrying about what they do *not* know and are unable to control. For other patients, uncertainty is associated with unbearable anxiety, hopelessness and fear. They may become preoccupied with '*what if*' thoughts about what might go wrong in the future. Some patients begin living their lives '*as if*' the worst has already happened.

For patients who are struggling to come to terms with uncertainty, it can be helpful to encourage them to face their fears, with a sensitive, open discussion about their specific anxiety-provoking thoughts. For example, a patient who fears dying may be afraid of future pain, or may be more concerned about the welfare of their loved ones after their death.

> "What is it about this that makes you feel so anxious?"

> "If that did happen, what would be the worst part about it for you?"

> "What do you imagine happening that causes you so much distress?"

The next stage may be to evaluate how realistic and helpful they are and to look for a more balanced view of the future:

> "Is this the most likely or realistic possibility? Is there any other way to view the situation?"

Strategies for managing uncertainty

Identify coping strategies for dealing with potential problems

Spend time with patients discussing and planning how they could cope if the worst really did happen. Ask the patient how they might cope with each feared possibility (switch '*What if...?*' thoughts to '*Then what...?*' plans).

Increase the patient's sense of control over life

Encourage patients to focus on aspects of their life that they genuinely have the power to change (e.g. how they spend their time each day), rather than continually focusing on areas they are powerless to control (e.g. what might happen in the future). This may include increasing time spent with family and close friends, or undertaking other enjoyable or meaningful activities.

Acceptance of uncertainty as a normal part of life

Life is *always* filled with uncertainty. By focusing on the worst possible outcome and behaving '*as if*' this is the most likely outcome, or '*as if*' the worst has already happened, the patient's life becomes filled with negative thoughts, feelings and unhelpful behaviours, which simply compound their problems.

Case Example 16.4: Managing uncertainty

Vanessa is a 45 year old woman who developed a malignant breast lump. The lump was successfully excised and subsequent scans revealed that there was no evidence of spread of the disease. One year later, Vanessa is well, with no signs of a recurrence. However, she remains preoccupied and anxious that the cancer could return.

Vanessa I can't stop worrying about the future. I keep thinking, *What if it comes back?* or *What if they can't treat it next time?* I know I am well now and I am so grateful, but I just wish I could feel more relaxed about the future.

GP What would you need to feel more relaxed about the future?

Vanessa I just need to be sure that the cancer won't come back.

GP You would like to feel certain that the cancer will never come back?

Vanessa Yes, although I know that is impossible. No-one can ever say that for sure.

GP I think you are probably right. No-one can ever be 100% sure about *anything* in the future. What is it about knowing for certain that would help you feel better?

Vanessa I would know that I could control things again.

GP What kinds of things would you like to have more control over?

Vanessa I could put my effort into continuing my life, by carrying on working, spending time with my children.

GP Are you concerned about losing control over these areas of your life?

Vanessa When I'm really anxious, I just think, *I know it's all going to come back* and I keep thinking about all these things that I will miss out on.

GP Are you doing these things less often than you used to?

Vanessa I suppose I am. I mean, what's the point of putting effort into working or building up my life, if it will all be taken away from me by the cancer?

GP It sounds like you are saying that you sometimes worry about your future health and think, *I know the cancer is going to come back,* which makes you feel very anxious. And you react by reducing some activities, because it seems pointless to do them if you will develop cancer in the future. Is that right?

Vanessa Yes it is. I hadn't really thought of it like that before.

GP What do you make of it now? Are there any ways that this pattern is unhelpful to you?

Vanessa Well yes, because it means that I am cutting down the things that are actually really important to me.

GP All this worrying might actually be getting in the way of you doing the things that are important to you. Supposing the cancer did come back

> eventually. How would you want to look back at your life between now and then? Do you think you would want to have spent most of that time worrying about the future?
>
> **Vanessa** No, not at all. I would probably want to think that I had enjoyed my life. I would want to have spent as much quality time as possible with my family. I wouldn't want to have spent all my time worrying about the future.
>
> **GP** What could you do differently, that might help you more?
>
> **Vanessa** I suppose I could try to focus on doing the things that really matter. Like spending time playing with my children and talking to my husband.

Changes in physical appearance

Many physical illnesses involve changes in appearance, which can cause a great deal of distress for some patients. If patients associate their changes in appearance with a loss of their personal worth or value, they are likely to experience a loss of self-esteem and a lowering of mood. The negative perception may result from patients' beliefs about changes in the opinion of others or it may result from their view of themselves. These negative self-views can be addressed directly using cognitive restructuring techniques. Behavioural experiments are also an effective means of reinforcing new, more helpful beliefs.

Case Example 16.5: Coping with changes in physical appearance

Reginald is a 76 year old widower who lives in a residential home. He has been diabetic for many years and suffers from vascular disease. He recently underwent a below-knee amputation. Reginald is well known for being a jovial man, who is well liked and sociable in the residential home. However, since his operation, he has become increasingly morose and withdrawn. During a visit, Reginald's GP spends a few minutes discussing his change in mood since the amputation:

Thoughts I look awful and others will not want to spend time with me. They will think I am not the same person any more – not 'whole'.

Feelings Sad

Behaviour Avoids social situations
Spends long hours alone in his room

Reginald's behavioural experiment planning chart:

What am I going to do? (What, where, when…?)	Attend the weekly in-house bingo evening. Invite a few old friends to join me.
What do I predict will happen?	My friends will react differently to me. They will seem uncomfortable and avoid looking at me. Some might make an excuse not to come or may sit elsewhere.
What problems might arise with this plan?	I might feel too tired or in too much pain to go.
How could these problems be overcome?	I will take my pain medication and have a brief nap during the afternoon beforehand.
What happened when I tried the experiment?	Everyone seemed very pleased to see me. A couple of people said that I looked very 'well.' No one tried to avoid me. Several people made a point of coming over and saying they were pleased to see me.

What have I learned from this experiment?

People don't necessarily think less of me for physical changes. Everyone changes in appearance with time for many reasons. This doesn't change me as a 'person'.

Coping with unpleasant physical symptoms

People with chronic disease may experience a wide variety of physical symptoms, including pain, dizziness, tinnitus, gastrointestinal symptoms, chronic cough or breathlessness. Some symptoms can be alleviated through the use of appropriate medication. However, many symptoms are difficult to eliminate entirely, and other symptoms may even be *caused* by the side-effects of drug therapy.

General strategies for coping with unpleasant physical sensations include:
- *Reduce self-focus*: reduce the amount of attention directed towards internal bodily processes. This can make physical sensations and symptoms seem less intrusive and unpleasant.
- *Distraction*: this can take the mind away from powerful unpleasant physical or emotional experiences.
- *Activity scheduling:* increase activities which are enjoyable or which give life a sense of meaning.
- *Graded exercise:* gradually build up exercise levels to increase fitness, improve mood and overcome fatigue and tiredness.
- *Relaxation:* decrease background levels of anxiety and tension.

- *Mindfulness* (see *Chapter 11*): can reduce the impact of unpleasant physical symptoms by encouraging patients to view them as simply one part of their experience.
- *Identify and treat underlying emotional disorders*: e.g. depression, anxiety or panic disorder.

Breathlessness in respiratory conditions

Breathlessness is a common symptom in conditions such as chronic obstructive pulmonary disorder (COPD). Some people will be able to tolerate this sensation whereas others find it extremely frightening and distressing. Patients can become extremely anxious and panicky about breathing difficulties and this may be associated with increased use of medical services.

Strategies for managing breathlessness include:
- Identifying catastrophic thoughts about breathlessness such as, *"I'm going to suffocate and die"* and looking for a balanced alternative perspective using guided discovery or a thought record.
- Giving clear explanations about anxiety and how it can also produce feelings of breathlessness which can worsen the sensation as a vicious cycle.
- Making a list of reassuring statements such as, *"This is frightening but I've coped with it many times before".*
- Building fitness and exercise tolerance through graded exercise or a pulmonary rehabilitation programme.
- Reducing safety behaviours such as over-use of inhalers when not required.
- Pursed lip breathing: start by relaxing the neck and shoulder muscles. Then take in a normal slow breath for a count of 2 through your nose. Finally, breathe out slowly through pursed lips for a count of 4. Repeat for a few minutes.
- Distraction.
- Increasing positive and meaningful activities and social interaction.

Key learning points

- The five areas of the CBM provide a useful structure to discuss psychological, emotional and behavioural aspects of chronic physical disease.
- Your aim is to help the patient to understand and manage their condition better themselves, and to improve their quality of life, independence and enjoyment, despite the presence of physical disease.
- A key focus is to increase functioning in valued life areas. Behavioural activation and activity scheduling are some of the most effective and useful ways of improving mood and reducing the emotional distress associated with physical health problems.
- Increase the patient's sense of control by encouraging them to make changes in areas of their lives that they genuinely have the power to influence.
- Try not to over-reassure anxious patients. Managing uncertainty about the future involves empathic listening to identify the patient's specific fears and then seeking ways to help them manage these negative thoughts, using thought records as well as looking for ways to cope if the worst really did happen (*'Then what...?'* planning).
- It will also help to provide clear explanations for all symptoms, including those caused by emotional factors such as anxiety. Make the explanation 'empowering' by including information that will help the patient to manage the symptom when it arises.
- Effective strategies for coping with unpleasant physical sensations include distraction, activity scheduling, mindfulness, relaxation and reducing focus on internal sensations.
- Remember to screen for depression and anxiety disorders, which are more common in patients with physical disorders but are underdiagnosed and undertreated.

Chapter 17

Functional somatic disorders

Chronic pain

What is chronic pain?

Chronic pain refers to pain that persists for at least 3 months after the usual recovery period for illness or injury. It can develop gradually as part of a chronic condition or be triggered by an acute injury. The pain does not respond well to usual treatments and causes tremendous suffering and a marked reduction in a patient's wellbeing and quality of life.

Chronic pain is an important primary care problem: 60% of patients with chronic pain visited their GP 2–9 times in the previous 6 months and 11% saw their GP at least 10 times (Breivik *et al.*, 2006). Musculoskeletal conditions are the most common cause of chronic pain in primary care, but it can be associated with many other conditions (*Box 17.1*).

Box 17.1

Common conditions associated with chronic pain

- Musculoskeletal conditions (e.g. arthritis, neck and back pain, fractures, sprains)
- Localised or regional pain problems (e.g. chronic pelvic pain, prostatitis, non-cardiac chest pain)
- Widespread pain syndromes (e.g. fibromyalgia, inflammatory or autoimmune conditions)
- Neuropathic pain (e.g. diabetic neuropathy, post-herpetic neuralgia, nerve injury, complex regional pain syndrome)
- Neurological conditions and headache (e.g. migraine, trigeminal neuralgia, tension-type headache)
- Other physical conditions causing persistent pain (e.g. cardiac disease, cancer)

Who gets chronic pain?

Certain groups of individuals are more likely to develop chronic pain or disability following an acute injury. Psychosocial barriers to recovery may be associated with poor outcomes including increased pain, long-term disability and worklessness (Hasenbring, 2012) (*Box 17.2*).

Box 17.2

Psychosocial barriers to recovery in acute back pain (Hasenbring *et al.*, 2012)

- Poor perceptions of general health
- Beliefs that pain and activity are harmful and avoiding activity will help recovery (fear avoidance)
- Catastrophising thinking styles and psychological distress
- Pain or illness behaviours such as extended rest
- Depression, low mood and social withdrawal
- History of back pain, time off; financial incentives
- Workplace factors such as job stress, physically demanding job, lack of co-worker support, job dissatisfaction and employer attitudes
- Stressful life events

Development of chronic pain

In chronic pain, the body's pain system may not function correctly, leading to persistence of pain despite the lack of ongoing injury or tissue damage. This can be explained by the gate control theory of pain (*Box 17.3*) and wind-up phenomenon (*Box 17.4*).

Box 17.3

Gate control theory of pain

The gate control theory (Melzack & Wall, 1965) suggests that the perception of pain is affected by the interaction between different neurons. This helps to explain how emotional and behavioural factors can influence the experience of pain.

When an individual experiences tissue damage or injury, pain 'messages' flow along peripheral nerves to the spinal cord and brain. In the spinal cord, there are 'nerve gates' (in the dorsal horn) which can inhibit (close) or facilitate (open) nerve impulses from the body to the brain. The more open these 'gates' are, the more pain an individual experiences.

- Factors which open the gates and increase the perception of pain include negative emotions and behaviours (e.g. constant worrying about the pain, feeling depressed and social withdrawal).
- Factors which close the pain gates and reduce pain include positive emotions, attitudes and behaviours (e.g. feeling in control, managing stress, graded exercise and spending time with friends and family).

Box 17.4

Wind-up phenomenon

People with chronic pain often believe that experiencing pain indicates ongoing tissue damage and injury. This can lead to unhelpful behaviours such as excessive rest to try to eliminate or avoid pain.

'Wind-up phenomenon' (Mendell & Wall, 1965) helps to explain why chronic pain may continue to get worse even without further injury or damage to the body. When people experience persistent pain, the nerves transmitting the painful impulses to the brain become 'trained' to deliver pain signals better. The intensity of the pain signals becomes greater and the perception of pain increases, even though the injury or illness is not changing. At this point, pain can be viewed as 'chronic' and is no longer helpful as a signal of illness.

CBT model of chronic pain

Typical thoughts in chronic pain

Patients with chronic pain typically hold a wide range of negative health beliefs and unhelpful thinking styles, including the following.

- Pain catastrophising: "*This pain is unbearable! I cannot cope with it.*"
- Belief that activity is dangerous: "*If my pain increases I must be doing permanent damage. It is better to rest when I feel any pain.*"
- Constant thinking and worrying about pain: "*The pain is so severe there must be something serious wrong with me.*"
- All or nothing thinking: "*I must be completely free of pain to feel better.*"
- Self-criticism and low self-esteem: "*Having this pain means I am weak, incompetent or unlovable.*"
- Thoughts about being out of control: "*Nothing helps to manage my pain.*"

Feelings in chronic pain

Patients with chronic pain often feel depressed, anxious about the future, experience a loss of enjoyment in their daily activities and may feel hopeless or helpless in the face of unremitting, intolerable pain. They may also feel tense, irritable and angry about their pain. These negative emotions are likely to lead to increased pain as a vicious cycle.

Physical symptoms

Chronic pain is associated with many types of physical discomfort including headaches, back pain, muscular pain, abdominal and pelvic pain. Other associated physical symptoms include:

- weakness and stiffness (often due to lack of activity)
- tension and anxiety-related symptoms; poor sleep
- lethargy and fatigue

- side-effects of medication
- weight gain due to inactivity and over-eating.

Behavioural changes

'Pain behaviours' are usually designed to either alleviate or prevent pain, or to gain support by informing others that the individual is suffering. In chronic pain, these behaviours often worsen the pain as a vicious cycle.
- Reduced activity and excessive resting in order to avoid pain.
- Social isolation and withdrawal.
- Poor pacing of activity with 'boom–bust' behaviour patterns.
- Sighing, groaning, grimacing on movement, limping, using walking sticks, wheel chairs or other physical aids, such as cervical collars.
- Talking about the pain excessively.
- Over-reliance on pain medication.
- Dissociating from self so as not to feel the pain.
- Taking on a 'sick role' in the family.

Environmental factors

Relevant psychosocial factors in chronic pain include:
- the social impact of chronic pain (e.g. loss of job / social status, financial difficulties)
- interpersonal factors (e.g. increased stress and pressure on families, altered relationships with others)
- background environmental / social difficulties (e.g. dissatisfaction with work, relationship problems)
- relevant past experiences of illness (in self and others)
- attitudes and relationships with health professionals.

Case Example 17.1: Fibromyalgia

Nisha is a 43 year old woman with widespread pain and extreme tiredness. She was diagnosed with fibromyalgia last year. She experiences aches, pains and burning sensations throughout her body, particularly her back and neck. She feels very stiff and finds it difficult to get going in the mornings. She also has periods of extreme fatigue that leave her unable to do anything at all.

The pain initially started when she had been under a lot of stress at work as a marketing director. She was working late nights and also dieting and exercising heavily to try to lose weight. She has now stopped working completely and reduced her exercise but finds that the pain and tiredness have not improved. She takes regular painkillers but they make her very drowsy. She has had several courses of physiotherapy, which helped a bit, but the pain does not completely go away and often returns a few months after finishing therapy.

Nisha and her GP complete the following CBM chart:

Thoughts and beliefs	Feelings
"I can't bear this terrible pain, it's ruining my life"	Irritable and frustrated
"The pain means my body is being damaged"	Low and worried
"Things will only get worse in the future"	
Behaviour	**Physical symptoms**
No longer going to work	Severe pain throughout body
Pushes herself hard on a 'good day' then pain is much worse afterwards (boom–bust)	Shooting, stabbing and burning pains
	Stiffness in the mornings
More isolated; reduced exercise and less physically active with children	Tiredness and episodes of extreme lethargy
Environment and background	
Left job to become a full-time mother – enjoys this but also misses her previous role	
Strained relationship with husband and kids due to low mood and irritability	

Vicious cycles in chronic pain

Many people with chronic pain have a great fear of experiencing pain. In order to avoid pain after an injury, they restrict their activities and may continue even after the original damage has resolved. This initially reduces pain but leads to a gradual loss of fitness, muscle strength and flexibility, and increased pain in the long term. Excessive focus on the pain also leads to increased anxiety and low mood, and an increased perception of pain as a vicious cycle (*Figure 17.1*).

Management of chronic pain

A CBT approach to chronic pain aims to shift the patient's focus from curing or eliminating pain to coping with the pain and improving quality of life, *despite the continued presence of pain*. It should involve a combined approach to treatment, which includes medical and psychological approaches. Any co-existing mood disorders, such as depression, should also be treated.

First steps – build a rapport

The first step in primary care is to build trust and improve relationships with patients. Ensure that you clearly acknowledge that the pain is real, extremely distressing and disruptive to the patient's daily life. Try to get to know the patient as a whole, learning about their family, hobbies or pets.

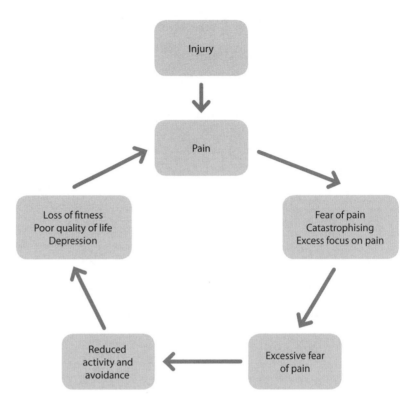

Figure 17.1: Vicious cycles in chronic pain

Take time to explore all aspects of the problem before offering any explanations or solutions. As with health anxiety (*Chapter 15*), it is helpful to begin by thoroughly reviewing the patient's physical symptoms in a longer initial consultation. Explain that discussing psychological factors does not mean stopping physical investigations or treatments when indicated.

Effective pain management may require a multidisciplinary approach, involving pain teams, primary care services and psychological support services. Remember to make early referrals to local pain specialists and pain management programmes, where available.

Empowering explanations

Always give clear explanations for the cause of chronic pain, such as the gate control theory of pain. This can help provide a rationale for a broader approach that includes the role of thoughts, emotion and behaviour in improving the patient's quality of life. You may also find it helpful to discuss the difference between 'hurt' and 'harm' and remind the patient that increased pain does not necessarily indicate further damage or worsening of the injury ('wind-up phenomenon').

From *theory* to *practice*...	Explain the difference between 'pain' and 'suffering' to help provide a rationale for increasing positive activities in patients with chronic pain.
	'Pain' represents their individual level of subjective discomfort. Remind the patient that it may not be possible to eliminate chronic pain completely and trying to do so may have unhelpful negative consequences that only worsen pain over time.
	In contrast, 'suffering' is the negative impact on an individual's life caused by the pain. It is often more helpful to focus on alleviating suffering rather than simply 'getting rid of' pain. This may involve making long-term choices to live in positive ways despite the pain.

Review and summarise the notes

For patients with long-standing chronic pain, it may be helpful to review their notes and write a summary of their key problems. This enables health professionals to make more informed decisions about medical care and can save a great deal of time and effort in the long term. The process may also reveal repetitive patterns of illness behaviour.

Using a pain diary

A pain diary can be used to record a patient's pain levels during a typical week (*Figure 17.2*). This can also be used to link pain to specific emotional or behavioural factors.

Date/time	What were you doing?	How severe was the pain? (rated 0–100)	How did you feel at this time? (e.g. angry, sad, anxious)	What did you do to cope with the pain? (How severe was the pain after this?)
Tuesday 10 a.m.	Watching TV	70	Fed up	Took pain killers Went to sleep (50)
Wednesday 1 p.m.	Making lunch	80	Anxious	Took pain killers Phoned a friend (60)

Figure 17.2: Pain diary

Behavioural strategies for managing chronic pain

Paced activity. Paced activity involves sticking to a planned baseline activity level until the patient has improved control of the pain, and then gradually increasing activity levels as their stamina and muscle strength improve. The patient chooses a realistic starting point that enables them to carry out the activity on a daily basis, on both good and bad days, and then builds gradually upwards. During a flare-up of pain or illness, they can reduce the activity back to baseline, rather than complete rest, to regain control, and then return to building up activities once things have improved.

Graded exercise. Patients are encouraged to engage in gradually increasing levels of physical exercise. This builds physical stamina and strength and also develops confidence in their ability to be active without any catastrophe taking place. It should involve small steps and realistic goals (e.g. starting with 5–10 minutes of walking or gardening).

Goal setting and behavioural activation. Encourage patients to increase meaningful and enjoyable activities despite the pain. They should also reduce unhelpful behaviours such as the amount of time spent reading or talking about pain to others. Behavioural changes should be simple, realistic and achievable, and should be planned and agreed collaboratively with the patient.

Behavioural experiments. Unhelpful beliefs about pain can be tested out using behavioural experiments (see *Case Example 17.2*).

Case Example 17.2: Behavioural experiments in chronic pain

John is a 42 year old mechanic, who has experienced long-standing back and shoulder pain following an accident at work. He has not worked for over 2 years.

Thoughts	"When I get the pain, it is better to rest otherwise I might do even more damage."
	"I must be completely free of the pain before I can get on with my life."
	"Nothing will ever improve for me."
Feelings	Sad, low
	Angry
Behaviour	Off work; spends hours lying on the sofa watching TV
	Increasingly isolated from his friends
Environment	8 year old son having problems at school; some marital difficulties
	Financial strain due to long-term unemployment

John's behavioural experiment planning chart:

Thought to test: *"I must rest when I get the pain or I will cause more damage and make things worse."*

Alternative view: *"Pain is not dangerous. It is better to remain active."*

What am I going to do? (What, where, when...?)	*"Try continuing activity despite the pain and see what happens." "I will try doing something I enjoy for 20 minutes, such as one or two DIY jobs around the house."*
What do I predict will happen?	*"I will experience agonising pain after 5 minutes of activity. This will continue for at least a day afterwards."*
What problems might arise with this plan?	*"I might feel too tired or not in the right mood to do it."*
How could these problems be overcome?	*"I will plan to do this even if I am not in the right mood and see what happens."*
What happened when I tried the experiment?	*"The pain continued but did not get worse. I was able to get a few things done and felt pleased with myself. My mood seemed a bit better afterwards."*

What have I learned from this experiment?
"It can be a good thing to keep active. The pain may not be as bad as I expect. I can still get things done, even if I have the pain."

Cognitive strategies

Cognitive strategies in chronic pain include identifying, evaluating and reframing any negative, unhelpful or catastrophic thoughts about pain, 'dangers' of activity or negative views of the future (*Box 17.5*).

Other cognitive strategies include:
- distraction: focus mind away from negative thoughts or pain
- encouraging acceptance: learning to view pain as an unpleasant but potentially inevitable part of life, accepting that complete cure of pain is unlikely
- mindfulness and relaxation.

Physical / medical strategies

Relaxation techniques, such as deep breathing, progressive muscular relaxation, massage and yoga, can be useful to improve pain and sleep.

Box 17.5

Reframing unhelpful beliefs about pain

Unhelpful belief	Balanced, more helpful perspective
"I must be completely free of the pain to feel better"	*"I can live a meaningful life even if I am experiencing pain"*
"As soon as I feel the pain I should rest to avoid doing any further damage"	*"'Hurt' is not the same as 'harm', and does not mean I am doing more damage. Being willing to experience some discomfort in the short term can help me to build fitness and strength and may reduce pain in the long term, as well as improving my quality of life."*
"I can't cope with such terrible pain"	*"I can and do cope with the pain, I have learned many different ways to cope when it arises"*
"I brought this pain on myself; it's all my own fault"	*"The pain is a medical problem which is no-one's fault; it is more helpful to look at ways of how I can improve my life rather than constantly blaming myself"*

Chronic fatigue syndrome

CBT model of chronic fatigue syndrome

Physical symptoms

Chronic fatigue syndrome (CFS) involves persistent mental and physical fatigue and exhaustion that is not improved by rest or sleep, and is often triggered by minimal exertion. Other symptoms include headaches, unrefreshing sleep, poor concentration and memory, tender glands, frequent sore throats and muscle pain. These symptoms may fluctuate in severity and intensity and can vary widely between different individuals. They have a major impact on the patient's daily life.

Thoughts

Patients with CFS typically hold a number of unhelpful beliefs and thinking styles including:

- fear about activity making the symptoms worse: *"If I do the slightest thing I will get completely exhausted"*
- fear of symptoms and the impact on their lives: *"The tiredness is completely unmanageable"*
- perfectionist beliefs which lead to boom–bust behaviour patterns: *"I must finish this job completely before I take a rest"*

- excessive focus on symptoms results in a worsening of symptoms and leads to further avoidance.

Behaviour

Patients with CFS tend to reduce or avoid activity and rest excessively. This leads to reduced fitness and muscle strength which worsens lethargy and fatigue as a vicious cycle. As in chronic pain, many patients with CFS have 'boom–bust' activity patterns interspersed with prolonged periods of rest. This makes it difficult to maintain activity routines and results in a gradual loss of fitness over time (*Figure 17.3*). People may also reduce important and meaningful activities including work, leisure and social activities. Sleep difficulties are worsened by irregular sleep patterns including daytime naps.

Feelings

Patients with CFS may feel depressed, low and worried about the future. These negative emotions lower the pain threshold, worsen feelings of tiredness and lead to low motivation and reduced activity levels.

From *theory* to *practice*...	It can be helpful to discuss emotional aspects of the problem, for example, by asking: "It sounds as if CFS has changed your life quite a lot, how does that make you feel?"
	However, some patients with CFS find it difficult to discuss their emotions or hold negative beliefs about expressing or sharing emotions with others. If an individual seems resistant to discussing emotional aspects of the problem, follow their lead and simply focus more on discussing relevant behaviours and thoughts.

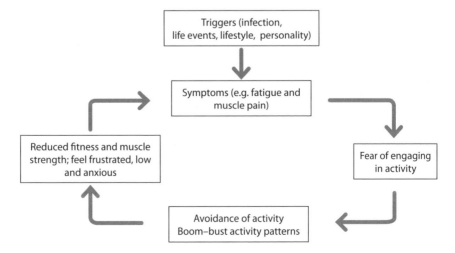

Figure 17.3: Vicious cycles in CFS

Environmental factors and triggers for CFS

Many patients believe that CFS symptoms are triggered by an illness such as a viral infection. However, there is no evidence that CFS is associated with any persistent infection and it is more likely that excessive resting following such an illness is to blame for the development of symptoms of fatigue.

People with CFS are more likely to have a hard-working and conscientious personality, and tend to have busy lifestyles with a lack of time for relaxation or enjoyable activities. Stressful life events such as the breakdown of a relationship, changing job or moving house can also trigger symptoms or make it more difficult to cope with symptoms of fatigue.

From *theory* to *practice*...

It is important to identify the patient's beliefs about the cause of their CFS symptoms. Ask the patient:

- What do you think caused your illness?
- What happened when the symptoms first started? What else was going on in your life?
- How did you cope with that problem?
- Could anything else be causing your symptoms now?

Make sure that you listen to their answers before jumping in with your own interpretation. Then provide an empowering explanation that encompasses their views and experience of the illness. Try not to directly challenge their views, even if you disagree with them, because this may cause a breakdown in your relationship. Rather than repeatedly debating the cause of the symptoms, focus on identifying any vicious cycles of thoughts and behaviour that may be maintaining or worsening symptoms.

Management of CFS

Engaging the patient

Being warm, empathic and using active listening will help to establish an effective relationship. Acknowledge that the patient's symptoms are real, distressing and having a major impact on their life. Take a holistic view of the cause of symptoms that avoids black and white views of the illness being either 'medical' or 'psychological' in nature. Collaboration and partnership are particularly important, ensuring that patients are encouraged to actively participate and set their own goals.

From *theory* to *practice*…	Be careful with your use of language and always try to use the patient's own words. For example, using the word 'tiredness' may provoke a highly negative reaction in a patient who differentiates strongly between the words 'fatigue' and 'tiredness'.

Behavioural strategies

Changing behaviour is one of the most important methods of improving CFS.

As with chronic pain, the aim is to establish a consistent pattern of activity and rest, rather than allowing activity to be planned according to the presence or absence of symptoms. Try to plan a minimum daily pattern of physical activity and aerobic exercise at a low level of intensity that can be kept up over time. The duration of the activity is gradually increased as the patient's strength and fitness improves. When the patient can cope with 30 minutes of low intensity activity, this can gradually be increased in intensity (e.g. walking more briskly).

Encourage the patient to view their symptoms as temporary and reversible, and resulting from their current lack of physical condition, rather than as signs of progressive pathology. Any mild or temporary increase in symptoms can be viewed as a normal reaction to an increase in physical activity, and the presence of symptoms should not prevent the patient from continuing to follow the activity plan.

Other behavioural strategies include:
- behavioural activation and goal setting: use activity diaries to plan increased meaningful and enjoyable activities
- behavioural experiments to test out unhelpful beliefs about the risks of activity
- establishing a sleep routine (see *Chapter 13*)
- graded exposure to situations that are being avoided due to anxiety.

Cognitive strategies

Cognitive techniques such as thought records and diaries can be used to address unhelpful thoughts and beliefs about activity. It is also important to identify and empathise with any anxiety about the cause of the symptoms. Strategies for managing health anxiety are covered in *Chapter 15*.

Case Example 17.3: Chronic fatigue symptoms

Katherine was a 40 year old accountant. She juggled a busy job and a hectic lifestyle, often working long hours alongside balancing her family commitments. She was also a keen runner who had completed several marathons in the past. One winter, she developed a severe flu-like illness which left her feeling exhausted for several weeks afterwards and she was frustrated to find that she was too tired to continue her schedule of long daily runs. Her tiredness and fatigue seemed to get worse and she developed exhaustion and flu-like symptoms after even minor activity, which was extremely disabling. When it had persisted for several months, she attended her GP. All tests were normal. Her GP completed the following CBM chart to understand Katherine's experience of fatigue:

Thoughts	Feelings
"Whenever I do too much my health completely breaks down" "It takes weeks to recover from even five minutes of exertion" "If I push on then I will pay for it in the long run"	Frustrated and fed up Low Guilty
Behaviour	**Physical symptoms**
Has given up running Rests or sits more often (finds standing tiring) Tries to 'push through' but feels exhausted after and has to rest (boom–bust) Continued to work but feels too tired for most social activities or hobbies	Extreme fatigue and flu-like symptoms after minor exertion Body aches all over Difficulty concentrating and disturbed sleep

Possible strategies for the GP:

- Highlight and discuss any vicious cycles that may be maintaining or worsening fatigue.
- Discuss alternatives to negative thoughts and highlight any unhelpful thinking styles such as catastrophisation.
- Use activity diaries and scheduling to plan enjoyable activities.
- Plan a behavioural experiment to find out what happens if she continues to be active for 5 minutes after experiencing symptoms of fatigue rather than resting immediately.
- Encourage gradual paced activity and graded exercise.
- Build a consistent sleep routine.

Irritable bowel syndrome

Irritable bowel syndrome (IBS) is a chronic non-inflammatory condition that causes abdominal pain, constipation, diarrhoea and abdominal bloating. Another common symptom is a feeling of incomplete evacuation after passing a stool.

IBS is not associated with any identifiable structural or biochemical change in the body. Patients with IBS should be assessed for more serious causes of their symptoms before a diagnosis of IBS is made. For example, weight loss, night pain and gastrointestinal blood loss should prompt further investigation.

CBT model of irritable bowel syndrome

Thoughts

Typical thoughts in IBS include:

- catastrophic thoughts about the meaning of symptoms: *"Maybe the pain is due to bowel cancer"*
- fears that symptoms are uncontrollable and may lead to embarrassment or shame in public: *"If I don't get to a toilet in time I might soil myself"*
- excessive focus on and awareness of symptoms
- beliefs that the body should be completely regular: *"I should open my bowels every day at the same time and produce a 'perfect' stool, otherwise there must be something wrong".*

Feelings

Catastrophic thoughts and fears in IBS cause a great deal of anxiety, which worsens bowel symptoms as a vicious cycle.

Behaviour

Typical behaviour in IBS is aimed at getting control over or eliminating unwanted symptoms. This includes:

- checking and testing for symptoms and signs of ill-health: this might involve checking stools for blood or for shape, colour or consistency, or measuring their abdomen for bloating
- constantly changing or monitoring dietary intake
- straining for long periods in order to open their bowels at the 'right' time or to ensure that the bowel is 'completely' empty
- avoidance of social situations for fear of embarrassment
- safety behaviours such as always carrying IBS medication, only visiting places with a toilet close at hand
- patients who are anxious about the cause of their symptoms may present frequently to health professionals requesting investigations and referrals to see a specialist.

Environment and background

IBS symptoms may be triggered by stressful life events and are often worsened by anxiety and stress.

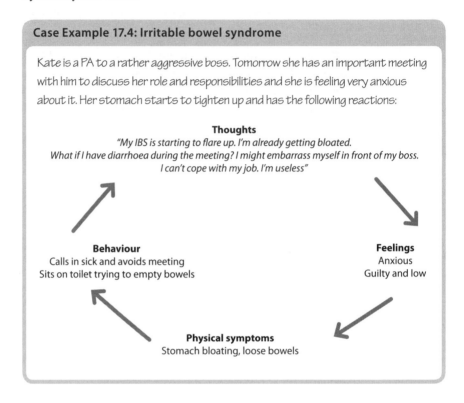

Case Example 17.4: Irritable bowel syndrome

Kate is a PA to a rather aggressive boss. Tomorrow she has an important meeting with him to discuss her role and responsibilities and she is feeling very anxious about it. Her stomach starts to tighten up and has the following reactions:

Thoughts
"My IBS is starting to flare up. I'm already getting bloated.
What if I have diarrhoea during the meeting? I might embarrass myself in front of my boss.
I can't cope with my job. I'm useless"

Behaviour
Calls in sick and avoids meeting
Sits on toilet trying to empty bowels

Feelings
Anxious
Guilty and low

Physical symptoms
Stomach bloating, loose bowels

Management of IBS

Effective health education

Talk through the patient's experience of their symptoms, using the five areas of the CBM as a template. Mapping the model to the patient's own experience of IBS symptoms will make your explanation far more compelling. An example of an empowering explanation for IBS is given in *Box 17.6*.

Box 17.6

Empowering explanation for IBS (adapted from Kennedy *et al.*, 2005)

Pain or discomfort in the abdomen, diarrhoea, flatulence and constipation occur to everyone at some stage. If you experience a particularly nasty bout of symptoms, this can make you vulnerable to experiencing these symptoms more and more.

IBS is a problem affecting the way the digestive system functions. It cannot kill you and is unlikely to get much worse. It normally comes and goes. For some

Box 17.6
Continued

people IBS will go away completely and for others it will never totally get better. Once you can accept the natural progress of IBS you can learn to cope with it. This will make it much easier to live with and may even stop it for good.

IBS is often worsened by stress. But this does not mean that IBS is all in the mind; far from it. IBS may have physical causes, but what you do, think and feel can maintain or aggravate many of these causes. IBS is likely to be connected to your lifestyle, to your level of anxiety and to the way you view the world and your IBS symptoms. By looking at and modifying what you feel, think and do, you will reduce the impact of IBS and lead a less restricted life.

It is OK to have IBS. It is nothing to be ashamed or apologetic about. There are lots of things you can do to reduce the effect it has on you.

It may also be helpful to discuss any health beliefs which may be contributing to the problem (see *Box 17.7*).

Box 17.7

Explanations for unhelpful health beliefs in IBS

Health belief	Empowering explanation
"I must pass a stool of the same shape and size every day."	It is normal for stools to vary in size, shape and consistency. This can be due to changes in diet, stress, anxiety or a change in environment such as travel abroad.
"By avoiding certain foods I will be able to control or avoid my symptoms."	IBS is caused by many factors including diet, emotions and behaviour. Special diets have been shown to have little benefit in IBS. Aim for a constant regular diet. Having a very restrictive diet or constantly worrying about your diet is likely to make matters worse.
"I must make sure that my bowel feels completely empty after each bowel movement. *I can only pass a stool if I keep straining."*	The feeling that your bowel is not completely empty is a common symptom in IBS. It does not necessarily mean that you must pass a stool. Continually straining when you don't need to pass a stool is likely to cause increased discomfort and worry.

Behavioural change techniques

It is helpful to use homework diaries and goal setting to plan changes in behaviour, including reducing unhelpful or safety behaviours and introducing alternative, more helpful coping strategies. Examples of useful goals might include:

- to reduce checking behaviour, such as checking stools for abnormalities
- to reduce straining and to only visit the toilet (to open bowels) when there is a definite urge to pass a stool
- to improve other toileting behaviour such as excessive wiping or time spent on the toilet, manual evacuation of bowels
- to gradually introduce foods that are being avoided if the diet is very restricted or the avoidance is causing disruption to the patient's life
- graded exposure to situations that are being avoided due to anxiety about symptoms, particularly important, meaningful and social activities, e.g. gradually returning to exercise or to places where a toilet is not immediately accessible.

Cognitive techniques

Useful cognitive techniques for IBS include:

- use of self-monitoring diaries to reduce examples of situations that they found difficult
- use of thought records to look for evidence for and against specific negative thoughts (e.g. "*If I can't get to the toilet within a few minutes I will have an accident*")
- distraction may be helpful to reduce symptom focusing
- distancing from negative or anxiety-provoking thoughts: switch from "*I can't cope with the pain*" to "*I'm having thoughts about not being able to cope with the pain*".

Managing anxiety about health

For anxious patients, accepting that they have IBS rather than anything more serious is an essential first step which is likely to lead to a reduction in anxiety and thus fewer symptoms. Strategies for managing anxiety about possible serious illness include health anxiety pie charts and the Theory A and Theory B method (see *Chapter 15*).

Key learning points

Summary of a general CBM for functional somatic disorders:

Thoughts and beliefs	Feelings
Fear and catastrophising about symptoms	Depression and low mood
Beliefs about the 'danger' of activity	Anxiety
Preoccupation and constant worry about symptoms; unhelpful health beliefs	Frustration and anger
Self-criticism and low self-esteem	
Behaviour	**Physical symptoms**
Reduced activity and excessive rest	Pain, weakness, stiffness
Avoidance; social isolation and withdrawal	Fatigue and tiredness
'Boom–bust' behaviour patterns	Poor sleep
Testing and checking aspects of health	Weight gain
Illness behaviours; poor sleep routines	
Environment and background	
Impact of symptoms (e.g. loss of job/social status, financial difficulties, stress and pressure on family)	
Development of symptoms may be associated with adverse life events	
Personality type, e.g. perfectionist, hard-working	
Relevant past experiences of illness (in self and others), attitudes and relationships with health professionals	

- When managing patients with functional somatic disorders, the main aim in primary care is to improve daily functioning by increasing the patient's engagement in meaningful and enjoyable activities.
- It is often more helpful to focus on behaviour than heavily emphasising emotional factors. Ask how the symptoms have changed their lives and what they are avoiding for fear of making symptoms worse or causing anxiety. Use a daily activity diary to monitor the patient's current helpful and unhelpful behaviour patterns. Encourage the patient to set achievable goals in line with their individual values and important life areas.
- Also key is to encourage paced activity and avoid boom–bust patterns of exercise or activity. Establish an achievable baseline of

daily activity and gradually build upwards. Help the patient plan ahead how they will cope with relapses or other potential problems.

- Discussing ways to manage general life stress using problem-solving, assertiveness (e.g. saying 'no' to excessive demands), time management, prioritisation of activities, building social networks and asking for support can help reduce background stress and make it easier to cope with challenging symptoms.

Chapter 18

Low self-esteem

What is low self-esteem?

In low self-esteem, people tend to view themselves as having little worth or value. It is associated with a range of other psychological difficulties and may be a symptom of underlying depression.

Self-confidence relates to people's beliefs about their ability to successfully achieve various goals, such as academic achievements, work success or relationships with others. In contrast, self-esteem reflects the overall opinion that people have of themselves as a person. This is not necessarily related to self-confidence or success. Thus, low self-esteem can occur in people who may outwardly appear to be very successful, and may drive some people towards continued high achievement in order to 'compensate' for their lack of self-worth.

The cognitive-behavioural model of low self-esteem

Thoughts and beliefs in low self-esteem

People with low self-esteem tend to be highly self-critical and hold a range of negative self-beliefs which exert a major influence on their lives and relationships with others. These include:

> "I'm worthless. I'm unlovable."

> "I'm inferior to others. I'm weak and stupid."

Unhelpful thinking styles in low self-esteem tend to involve a negative or biased view of the self:

- *Ignoring the positive*: ignore or discount praise, successes or strengths
- *Negative view of the self*: viewing self negatively, 'self-prejudice'; focus on mistakes, weaknesses and criticisms
- *Mind-reading*: negative perception of others' opinions and over-sensitivity to criticisms or disapproval from others
- *Self-blame*: taking excessive personal responsibility when things go wrong.

These negative thoughts may often represent underlying core beliefs and rules about the self (see *Chapter 10*).

Feelings

Low self-esteem is associated with a variety of negative feelings, including sadness and depression, anxiety, anger, guilt and shame.

Behaviour

People with low self-esteem tend to behave '*as if*' their negative self-beliefs are absolute fact. This destructive and self-fulfilling behaviour worsens low self-esteem as a vicious cycle, and may include:

- lack of assertiveness, trying to please others excessively, inability to say 'no' ("*I must do what others want, otherwise they will reject me*")
- underperformance and avoidance of challenges and opportunities ("*There is no point in trying – I am too stupid to succeed*")
- setting themselves up to fail ("*This proves I am completely useless*")
- perfectionism and over-work ("*Making a single mistake means I am a failure*")
- avoiding intimate relationships or ending up in abusive relationships ("*I am unlovable*")
- shyness, avoiding social situations ("*I am boring and inadequate*")
- difficulty making decisions ("*I always do the wrong thing*")
- poor self-care, using drugs, obesity ("*I am not worth taking care of*")
- excessive care with physical appearance ("*Looking attractive is the only way to be acceptable to others*").

Physical symptoms

Low self-esteem and its associated low mood can lead to physical symptoms such as muscle tension, tiredness and lethargy, sleep problems and changes in appetite and weight.

Environment and social factors

Experiencing social or environmental problems such as relationship problems, financial or economic difficulties, chronic stress or physical illness, can result in feelings of incompetence, inadequacy and low self-esteem. In this situation, tackling the underlying problem using problem-solving may be an important strategy (see *Chapter 9*). It is also often helpful to work concurrently on building self-esteem to help the person address their difficult life problems.

The development of low self-esteem

The negative ideas and beliefs in low self-esteem are learned from people's life experiences, including childhood difficulties and traumatic experiences during adulthood (*Box 18.1*). These experiences lead to the development of low self-esteem if people view them as a sign of *personal failure or inadequacy*, rather than as simply unfortunate events that could happen to anyone. Children are particularly likely to blame themselves for negative life events.

| Box 18.1 | **Negative life experiences associated with low self-esteem** |

Early or childhood experiences
- History of abuse or neglect (physical, sexual or emotional)
- Being bullied
- Excessive criticism, lack of affection or praise; unrealistic expectations from parents
- Perceived rejection or being different to others
- Low self-esteem, stress or emotional distress of parents

Later experiences
- Long-standing stress or hardship
- Abusive relationships
- Being bullied in the workplace
- Traumatic events (e.g. bereavements, assaults, accidents)
- Loss of status or role (e.g. unemployment, disability)
- Psychological or emotional disorders (e.g. depression, panic attacks)

Case Example 18.1: The development of low self-esteem

Gemma's story

Gemma was the daughter of a 17 year old single mother with little social support. Gemma's mother loved her daughter but struggled to cope with the demands of a young child and Gemma was fostered several times. She blamed herself for being abandoned by her mother believing, "It's my fault she left me because I'm worthless and unlovable". The constant changing of area and school left Gemma feeling insecure and unstable, and she became moody and sullen. Gemma rarely stayed long with the same family, and blamed herself for this: "No one wants me around for long – it must mean that I'm a really bad person". When Gemma was permanently adopted at the age of 11, she was mistrusting of her new family's affection and constantly expected to be rejected again. In adult life, Gemma found it difficult to trust others or to feel secure in loving relationships. She tended to choose partners who let her down and treated her with little care or respect. Even when people did care about Gemma, she found it difficult to believe or trust them.

Bobby's story

Bobby suffered from meningitis as a young child and developed mild hearing loss which was not picked up for some time. He was a boisterous child with a lot of energy. He struggled to hear the teachers at school and compensated by channelling his energy into rowdy behaviour. His academic performance dropped compared to his brothers and his teachers labelled him 'lazy' and 'attention-seeking'. Bobby's parents became frustrated with his behaviour and Bobby was continually in trouble. *"What's the point in trying?"* he thought, *"I'm just stupid".*

Overcoming low self-esteem

Overcoming low self-esteem involves developing a range of more helpful attitudes and behaviour including:

- a more balanced view of the self which includes both positive and negative aspects with increased self-acceptance ('warts and all')
- increased self-confidence and willingness to attempt and achieve goals; improved view of own skills, qualities and abilities
- increased sense of self-worth.

Discovering the internal bully

The negative, self-critical thoughts in low self-esteem can be compared to an internal bully. Like a nagging parent, these thoughts can be viewed as trying to *help*, by ensuring that the person does not make any mistakes. However, the constant criticism is likely to have a negative effect by undermining confidence and self-esteem.

The first step in making change is to recognise that the thoughts are present and may be damaging. One approach is to construct an image of the criticisms coming from a third person. This helps the patient to 'unhook' or disassociate from the thoughts, so that they are not immediately accepted as being absolute truth.

From *theory* to *practice*...

Ask a patient with low self-esteem to imagine their self-critical thoughts coming from an imaginary external figure. Encourage them to choose their own image, e.g. a small radio, or a gremlin or parrot sitting on their shoulder, shrieking loud, critical comments into their ear.

What kinds of things does the 'creature' say? What tone or voice or volume does it have? Is it fair or realistic?

Is this how you would talk to another person or child? Why not? Is there another way to get the same message across which is kinder and more compassionate?

The rational mind

Being rational involves looking at the *evidence* for a particular thought or belief rather than immediately assuming it is accurate or correct. Rather than being swayed by *emotional* evidence or reasoning (*It feels as if it must be true*), being rational involves taking time to carefully consider the situation and avoiding jumping to conclusions (see *Box 18.2*). This may include weighing up the pros and cons of any particular viewpoint or course of action before making a decision, and taking a broader or longer-term view of problems.

Box 18.2	**Questions to develop the rational perspective**
	• *"How do I know this is true? What is the evidence for and against this viewpoint?"*
	• *"How else could I view this situation?"*
	• *"What would I like to achieve in the long term?"*
	• *"What is the most important issue to me?"*
	• *"What would be the most helpful way to approach this situation?"*

The compassionate mind

Another key approach to overcoming low self-esteem is for people to learn to treat themselves with kindness and compassion (see *Box 18.3*). Developing the compassionate mind encourages people to become their own 'best friend'. Patients learn to support and reassure themselves, and to offer themselves the same kind, caring attitude which they often extend to others. Whilst it is pleasant to receive positive feedback from others, it is important not to depend entirely on others to maintain self-worth. Therefore, as well as learning to get support from others, people also need to learn how to give themselves an internal 'stroke' or 'hug'.

Box 18.3	**Questions to develop the compassionate mind**
	• *"What would you say to a close friend or family member if they were in the same situation? What might they say to you?"*
	• *"If you wanted to be kind to someone in a similar situation, what would you say?"*
	• *"How could you look at this situation without criticising or blaming yourself or others?"*
	• *"Are you remembering your qualities and achievements as well as the negatives or failures?"*
	• *"Are you expecting perfection from yourself? Is this fair or realistic?"*

Many people with low self-esteem are kinder, more diplomatic and less judgemental with others than with themselves. This is useful, because it means that people already possess the ability to be supportive and compassionate, and simply need to learn to apply these rules and communication styles to themselves as well.

Case Example 18.2: Developing the compassionate mind

Jessica is a 28 year old woman with low self-esteem who is highly self-critical and views herself as unattractive and of little worth. She was bullied at school for being overweight. The following dialogue illustrates a discussion between Jessica and her GP.

GP   *Could you give me an example of a recent situation where you were self-critical or negative about yourself?*

Jessica *Yes, last week. I forgot to record my boyfriend's favourite TV show. He said it wasn't a big deal but I felt so stupid.*

GP   *What thoughts went through your mind about yourself?*

Jessica *I couldn't even manage such a simple thing. I felt like such an idiot. My boyfriend would be better off with someone else. I'm not even attractive.*

GP   *I've written down all the things you said to yourself when you forgot to record the show: I'm stupid, I couldn't even manage such a simple thing, I'm an idiot, My boyfriend would be better off without me, I'm not attractive'. How does it make you feel to think these things?*

Jessica *I feel awful – really low and depressed.*

GP   *I think that's understandable, given all these critical thoughts that you are having. Supposing your best friend had forgotten to record a programme for her boyfriend, would you say those things to her? Would you tell her that she was 'stupid' and her 'boyfriend would be better off without her'?*

Jessica *No. No, I would never say that to anyone else.*

GP   *Why not?*

Jessica *It would hurt her feelings. It would be a nasty thing to say.*

GP   *What would you say to her instead?*

Jessica *I'd tell her that it's just a small mistake to make. She shouldn't beat herself up about it. Her boyfriend didn't care about it, so why should she?*

GP   *That sounds like very good advice. Supposing she keeps saying that she's stupid and that her boyfriend would be better off without her. If you wanted to be kind and supportive, what would you say?*

Jessica *I would tell her that she was great and that she shouldn't think so badly of herself.*

GP	How could you convince her of that?
Jessica	I could remind her of all the ways she's supported me in the past.
GP	That sounds really good. Do you think it might help her to tell her exactly what it is that you like about her?
Jessica	I could say that she is good fun to be with and she's always there when I need her.
GP	Excellent. Now, how could you apply all of that discussion to yourself?
Jessica	I can see that I talk to myself in ways that I would never use with anyone else.
GP	And if you wanted to give yourself the same support that you gave to your friend, what could you do?
Jessica	I suppose I could tell myself that I am not stupid and try to think up some positive things to say to myself too.
GP	It seems like you are already very good at being supportive and caring to other people. It might help you to use some of these skills with yourself too. Perhaps you could think about how you might do this over the next couple of weeks.
Jessica	It feels very strange but I will definitely think about it.

Countering negative thoughts and self-criticism

Using written thought records

Written thought records are a powerful way of overcoming low self-esteem by questioning the evidence for and against self-critical thoughts and finding a more balanced alternative viewpoint.

Case Example 18.2: *Continued*: using thought records to overcome self-critical thoughts

Jessica uses a thought record to test out one of her negative, self-critical thoughts:

Thought to test out	
"My boyfriend is better off without me."	
Evidence *for* the negative thought	**Evidence *against* the negative thought**
"I'm not as attractive as many other women."	"My boyfriend thinks I am attractive – he often says so."
"I make stupid mistakes like forgetting to record his programme."	"He enjoys my company. We have plenty of good conversations."

"I'm not as chatty or interesting as other people." *"I get quite depressed and low sometimes, which is difficult for him to be around."*	*"I am a good listener and he appreciates having someone to talk through his problems."* *"I am not always depressed – we do have fun together as well."* *"I am trustworthy and kind and would never deliberately do anything to hurt him."*
Alternative / balanced thought to replace the hot thought: *"My boyfriend loves me as I am – he doesn't want me to be any different. I have many good qualities and I contribute as much to our relationship as he does."*	

When a negative thought involves 'mind-reading', it is sometimes helpful for the patient to *ask the other person what they really think*. This is particularly helpful with close family members or partners, who may describe many of the patient's positive qualities. However, it can be counterproductive to ask a particularly critical partner or family member, who may reinforce the negative perspective.

From *theory* to *practice*…

When patients use negative, black and white thinking styles, such as *"I'm a complete failure"*, one way to broaden their perspective is to discuss this in terms of a rating scale or 'continuum' (Greenberger & Padesky, 1995a).

Ask the patient what each end of the scale should be, such as 'complete failure' at one end and 'complete success' at the other end:

Failure -- Success

Begin by discussing what it would mean to be a *complete failure*. Ask them to describe someone who had failed in every possible way. Make sure that the description is as extreme as possible. Would this person fail to dress themselves in the morning? Would they fail to prepare themselves food? What would their relationships be like with others? Is it possible for *anyone* to be a complete failure?

Next, ask the patient what a *complete success* would look like. Is it possible to succeed in every single way? How realistic is this? What effect might this have on relationships with others? What might they have to do to ensure success at all costs? Does this make them a nicer or more worthwhile person?

Finish by discussing a more balanced and realistic perspective. The reality is that everyone lies somewhere in between the two extremes. Ask the patient how they could apply this view to their own difficulties.

Identifying personal qualities

It is valuable for patients with low self-esteem to make a written record of positive achievements, personal qualities and strengths. The list should include a wide range of qualities (*Box 18.4*). It is often helpful for the health professional to spend a few minutes beginning the exercise with patients, and then encourage them to continue it for homework (see *Box 18.5*).

Remind patients to avoid black and white thinking about particular qualities. It is not necessary (or even possible) to be caring or supportive 100% of the time for these qualities to be valuable and important. People with low self-esteem will often initially find this exercise difficult and uncomfortable. They may react with a stream of negative thoughts that immediately discount any positive qualities (*"That's nothing special – everyone does that"*, *"I don't do that often enough"* or *"I should have done it better than that"*).

Box 18.4

Examples of personal qualities

Kind	Intelligent	Honest	Supportive
Interesting	Reliable	Caring (for others)	Caring (for self)
Punctual	Determined	Successful	Trustworthy
Friendly	Funny	Considerate	Likeable
Smart	Competent	Good listener	Thoughtful
Loving	Helpful	Brave	Enthusiastic

Box 18.5

Questions for identifying positive qualities

- *"What good qualities can you notice in yourself? Is there anything you like about yourself, no matter how small it may seem?"*
- *"What would someone who cares about you say that your strengths or positive qualities are?"*
- *"Think of one or two people who you like or respect. What do you value in them? Do you have any of these qualities?"*
- *"What achievements have you made in your life so far, however small or simple? This might include maintaining friendships, having a job, caring for others, or carrying out hobbies or interests."*
- *"What difficulties or obstacles have you coped with or overcome in your life? Did this involve qualities such as strength, courage or determination?"*

> **Case Example 18.2:** *Continued*: identifying positive qualities to boost self-esteem
>
> Jessica is encouraged by her GP to make a list of her qualities. She finds the exercise initially difficult but eventually she is able to come up with the following list:
>
> | Quality | Evidence that I have this quality |
> |---|---|
> | Considerate | "I remembered my friend Helen's birthday and sent her a nice card and present."
 "When my boyfriend was ill, I did all his shopping and cooked him a nice meal." |
> | Determined | "Even though I was teased at school, I still managed to pass my exams and went on to college."
 "I keep going to work, even when I feel depressed or low." |
> | Trustworthy | "My boyfriend has given me a key to his house because he trusts me."
 "Several of my friends have trusted me with personal information about themselves because they say I am a good listener (e.g. Jane, Helen)." |
> | Caring | "I take good care of my cat."
 "I often visit my parents to see how they are and try to do things to help them if I can." |
> | Skilled | "I can cook well, drive and swim."
 "I am learning to use a computer for work – it's not easy but I am improving." |
> | Likeable | "I have several friends who like me; I have known Helen for many years."
 "My boss seems to like me – he is always pleasant and polite." |

Positive diaries

Positive diaries can be used to encourage patients with low self-esteem to record evidence of achievements, personal qualities and praise from others. This written information is useful to call on when the patient is feeling low or discouraged, and has fallen into habitual self-critical thinking patterns. The diary should be completed on a daily basis over a period of months. It should also include many small examples of positive achievements, rather than waiting for 'major' events.

Case example 18.2: *Continued*: Jessica's positive diary

Date	What happened?	What positive quality / qualities does this indicate?
12th March	Tidied up my flat and did my washing	Care for myself
	Cooked nice dinner for myself	Competent
13th March	Invited to lunch with work colleagues	Likeable
	Finished my project at work and submitted report to boss	Reliable, competent
14th March	Went in to work, despite feeling fed up	Determined
	Phoned my sister to see how she is, although I felt tired after a long work day	Thoughtful, caring
15th March	Invited to lunch with work colleagues again	Likeable
	My friend Helen called for a chat and told me about some of her problems at work	Likeable, trustworthy, supportive, good listener

From *theory* to *practice*...

People with low self-esteem frequently focus on one minor problem or mistake and ignore all their positive qualities and achievements. However, no-one can be perfect! A visual way of illustrating this involves representing the individual as a large circle filled with dots and crosses:

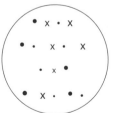

Each dot represents a success that the patient has achieved and each cross represents something that went wrong. By focusing on one small mistake (illustrated by a small cross) the patient is ignoring all their other achievements, which are still very much part of the whole.

A more realistic view accepts the presence of both successes and mistakes. *Everyone* makes mistakes sometimes and it is impossible to succeed at everything. Making a mistake or failing in some way does not indicate that the person is a *complete failure*. It simply indicates that the person is normal and human.

Changing unhelpful behaviour in low self-esteem

Increasing activity levels

Increasing activity is a useful method of improving mood for people who are experiencing low self-esteem. It may be helpful to use an activity chart to identify the patient's current activity levels and to plan future changes (see *Chapter 7*).

The patient should try to reduce self-defeating or unhelpful activities, such as excessive resting or withdrawal from others. It is helpful to take a step-by-step approach to increasing activities which are enjoyable, give the patient a sense of achievement and take into account the needs of the patient as well as others.

Behavioural experiments

Behavioural experiments can be used to boost self-esteem by undermining negative self-concepts and reinforcing positive self-beliefs.

Case Example 18.3: Using behavioural experiments to overcome low self-esteem

Example 1: Negative thought being tested: *"I made a mistake at work – this means I am no good at my job"*

What could I do to test this thought in practice? (What, where, when…?)	*"I could ask my boss for feedback on my performance."*
What do I predict will happen?	*"She will say that my performance is very poor."*
What problems might arise with this plan?	*"I might feel too nervous to ask her."*
How could these problems be overcome?	*"I could plan out what I want to say in advance and how I will respond if she is very negative."*
What happened when I tried the experiment?	*"She said that she was happy with my work in general."*

What have I learned from this experiment?

"Maybe I am more competent than I thought. Making one small mistake may not be a major disaster."

Example 2: Negative thought being tested: *"Jane doesn't like me because she didn't reply to my e-mail"*

What could I do to test this thought in practice? (What, where, when...?)	*"I could phone Jane and ask her if she would like to meet up sometime soon."*
What do I predict will happen?	*"She will ignore my call or make an excuse not to meet up."*
What problems might arise with this plan?	*"She might be out when I call or not answer the phone."*
How could these problems be overcome?	*"If she is out, I can leave a message on her answer-phone asking her to call me back."*
What happened when I tried the experiment?	*"She was out when I called, but she rang back the next day and said she was pleased that I had called and invited me out. She said she has been very busy with work recently."*

What have I learned from this experiment?

"Maybe Jane does like me – she was just busy. I jumped to the worst conclusion about why she hadn't replied to my e-mail."

Developing assertiveness

Developing assertiveness involves learning to ensure that our own needs, feelings or rights are taken into consideration by others, *without* becoming aggressive, demanding or rude, and whilst maintaining respect for other people (*Box 18.6*). This is likely to result in an increase in self-confidence and self-esteem and an increase in respect from others.

Box 18.6	**Aspects of assertiveness**

- Able to see both sides of a situation and recognise the needs and rights of everyone involved
- Take responsibility for our own actions
- Ask for what we want, directly and openly, but without undermining others or violating their rights
- Ensuring our needs are taken into account but not purely focusing on or getting our own way; being prepared to negotiate or compromise if necessary
- Recognise that we have something to contribute to others, irrespective of the opinions of others
- Take responsibility for fulfilling our own needs

Making assertive statements and requests

There are four stages of expressing assertive statements:
1. Describe the problem clearly and objectively: this should be an objective, factual description of what problem has triggered the discussion.
2. Explain how the situation makes you feel: use 'I' to describe how the situation affects you personally, taking responsibility for the way you feel, rather than blaming others.
3. Express your needs and what you would like to achieve.
4. Explain the consequences of making the change: include the specific positive outcome of making the change, both for you and the other person, as well as the consequences of failing to change.

It is often helpful for patients to plan out ways to increase their assertive behaviour in advance by rehearsing or writing down what they plan to say.

Case Example 18.4: Making assertive statements

The following statement includes all four stages of assertiveness:

*"In a recent report on my work, I was described as lacking commitment and dedication **[event]**. I feel rather upset and frustrated by this because I have been working very hard recently on several projects **[feeling]**. I would like to find out why I was described in this way because I believe I am hard-working and committed and would like to ensure that others are also aware of this **[need]**. This will help motivate me to continue to do my best in this job **[consequence]**."*

Learning to say 'no'

Becoming more assertive may involve learning when to say 'no'. The principles of saying 'no' are as follows:
- be honest and direct about saying 'no', while remaining courteous and polite rather than being blunt or rude
- communicate the reasons for saying 'no' in simple, concrete terms
- avoid apologising or giving complex, elaborate reasons for saying 'no'
- remember that everyone has the right to say 'no' if they don't want to do something.

The 'broken record' technique can also be a useful strategy for saying 'no' (see *Case Example 18.5*).

Case Example 18.5: Using the broken record technique to promote assertiveness

Christine is a single parent who relies heavily on her mum, Joyce, to help out with her son. Joyce is 59 and has recently started a part-time job as a catering manager in a school kitchen. Joyce is finding the work rewarding but busy and has set aside the evening to plan her menus for the next week.

Christine Would you be able to baby-sit for me tonight? I've been invited to a concert.

Joyce I'm sorry. I can't help tonight as I need the evening to catch up on some paperwork.

Christine Oh, please. It will be such a good show. I'll make it up to you.

Joyce I'm afraid I can't help tonight – I'm catching up on some paperwork.

Christine You could do that any time. I never get out much these days. Surely you don't want me to miss out on this?

Joyce You know that I love to help wherever I can, but I just can't help tonight. I'm too busy with paperwork.

Dealing with criticism

It is important for patients with low self-esteem to learn to cope with other people's defensive or critical reactions to their attempts at assertiveness. These responses can be very hurtful, particularly if they contain a small grain of truth. Becoming defensive in response to criticism is usually counterproductive because it deflects attention away from the most important issues and may lead to an unhelpful debate or argument.

A more helpful approach is to calmly acknowledge the other person's perspective. This may encourage them to be more flexible and helpful in return, and helps to maintain focus on the most important issues. Then take time to respond in a way that calmly and clearly asserts your own perspective.

Key learning points

Summary of the CBM for low self-esteem:

Thoughts and beliefs	Feelings
View self as having little worth or value; self-criticism ("*I'm hopeless and stupid*")	Depression, sadness and low mood
Mind-reading and oversensitivity to criticism ("*People don't think I've got any value*")	Guilt and shame
	Irritability and anger
Self-blame ("*I always say the wrong thing*")	Anxiety
Behaviour	**Physical symptoms**
Lack of assertiveness	Physical tension
Under-performance and avoidance of challenges	Tiredness and lethargy
Perfectionism and over-work	Poor sleep
Avoidance of intimate relationships or social situations	
Difficulty making decisions	
Environment and background	
Early childhood experiences predispose to low self-esteem (e.g. abuse, neglect, critical parenting, rejection or bullying)	
Social or environmental problems undermine self-esteem (e.g. relationship, work or financial problems, chronic stress or physical illness)	

- People with low self-esteem view themselves as having little worth or value as a person. However, people who seem to be outwardly highly successful may still suffer with low self-esteem.
- Behaving 'as if' beliefs about being worthless, stupid or inferior to others are true tends to worsens low self-esteem as a vicious cycle.
- Encourage patients to develop a rational and compassionate view of themselves and to accept that being imperfect and fallible is a normal human trait.
- Strategies to build self-esteem in the GP consultation include keeping a 'positive' diary which records daily evidence of an individual's qualities and achievements.
- Changing behaviour is also important. Use a behaviour monitoring chart or ask the patient to keep a diary of unhelpful and helpful behaviour patterns. Next plan a behavioural experiment to try an alternative behaviour that may build self-esteem.

Chapter 19

Managing 'heartsink'

What is 'heartsink'?

'Heartsink' is a subjective negative reaction within a health professional when faced by a particular patient, situation or even colleague. The clinician might feel low, depressed, anxious, angry, frustrated or guilty.

GPs describe a remarkably broad range of patient groups as associated with a heartsink reaction (*Box 19.1*). However, the reality is that different GPs will experience heartsink in varying situations. Whilst some patient groups are undoubtedly more challenging to manage in primary care, the development of heartsink depends upon the reaction of a particular GP to that patient or situation, rather than being an inherent characteristic of any particular patient.

The term 'heartsink patient' is commonly used but is inaccurate and may be viewed by patients as derogatory. Blaming the patient for the problem is also likely to prevent health professionals from seeking more effective personal strategies for managing the situation.

Box 19.1	**Patient groups commonly described as 'heartsink' (Steinmetz & Tabenkin, 2001)**

- Violent, aggressive or verbally abusive
- Complaining, never satisfied, demanding
- Manipulative, lying
- Lacking respect for doctor's knowledge / experience
- Impossible to help
- Litigious
- Uncooperative with recommended treatments or suggestions
- Unrealistic expectations from clinicians or the NHS
- Unresolved, repeated complaints or presentations ('frequent attenders')
- Multiple complaints – presenting with a 'shopping list'
- Complex or vague presentations, e.g. everything hurts or tired all the time
- Talkative, rambling – 'difficult historians'
- High levels of anxiety; difficult psychiatric cases
- Drug addicts

Who gets heartsink?

Certain factors (*Box 19.2*) and personality traits (*Box 19.3*) are associated with the more frequent experience of heartsink in general practice consultations.

Box 19.2	**Factors associated with GPs reporting greater numbers of 'heartsink patients' (Butler & Evans, 1999; Mathers *et al.*, 1995)**
	• Less experienced doctors • Lack of training in communication skills • Lower job satisfaction • Greater perceived workload • Lack of postgraduate qualifications • Underlying personal emotional problems (e.g. depression or anxiety)

Box 19.3	**Personality traits and associated beliefs likely to increase heartsink experiences**

	• Highly critical, judgemental or intolerant character (of self or others)
	   – patients should only present with 'genuine' medical problems
	   – that patient is simply a hypochondriac, attention-seeker
	• High levels of personal anxiety and difficulties coping with uncertainty
	   – I need to be 100% certain that I haven't missed anything serious before I can relax
	   – making any kind of mistake is a major disaster
	• Being overly nice or needing to be constantly liked by others
	   – my patients must all like me; otherwise I'm not being a good doctor
	   – patients must be given as much time as they need
	• Defensive personality or difficulty coping with criticism
	   – I must never be seen to be wrong
	   – patients should only come to see me if they will follow my advice

From *theory* to *practice*...	Reflect on the patients who are most likely to generate your own heartsink reactions. Can you identify any personality traits and associated clusters of beliefs which might result in your responses? How are these beliefs *helpful* to you? How might they be *unhelpful* or result in heartsink reactions?

Taking responsibility for heartsink reactions

General practice involves caring for a wide range of patients with varied health needs that span physical, psychological and social dimensions. Such patients have varied personalities, health beliefs, behaviours and ways of interacting with health professionals. It is therefore necessary to develop effective strategies for coping with patients and situations that we may find challenging.

The first step is to take responsibility for our own reactions. There is no way to directly change another person, but by changing our own unhelpful thoughts or behaviours, we can influence the *interaction* or *relationship* between GP and patient. This will help GPs feel more in control and reduce the sense of anxiety and stress associated with the situation.

The CBM approach to heartsink

The CBM provides a useful framework to understand heartsink reactions. The aim is not to eliminate negative thoughts or feelings about individual patients, but to learn to manage these reactions more effectively. This helps to ensure that caring for patients does not exert an undue emotional toll, and prevent the development of stress, depression or burnout. Managing heartsink reactions can also improve the clinical management of certain patients, which may be adversely affected by a GP's negative emotions such as anger or anxiety.

Feelings associated with heartsink

Common emotions that arise during heartsink reactions include guilt, anger, frustration, irritation, anxiety, sadness or depression. Remember that perceiving increasing numbers of 'heartsink patients' can also be a sign of a more serious underlying emotional disorder, such as anxiety or depression, which should be addressed directly.

Thoughts

The next step is to identify the thoughts and beliefs that underpin the negative feelings in heartsink reactions (*Box 19.4*).

Behaviour

Understanding and changing unhelpful behaviour can be one of the most effective methods of improving heartsink reactions (*Box 19.5*).

Box 19.4

Questions to identify key negative automatic thoughts

- What goes through my mind when I am faced by this patient?
- What is the worst bit about this?
- What does the situation say about me as a doctor or as a person?
- Am I concerned that something might happen? What would be the worst thing?
- What do I believe the patient thought or felt about me in that situation? What does that mean to me?

Box 19.5

Identifying and understanding behavioural reactions

- Identifying helpful and unhelpful behaviour:
  - How do I react to this patient? Do I behave differently with them than others?
  - Do I know anyone else who might react differently? What would they do?
- Understanding the thoughts / beliefs which drive the behaviour:
  - What makes me react that way? What might happen if I didn't?
- Exploring the impact of the behaviour:
  - How does this behaviour affect me or others (patients, colleagues, family, friends…)?
  - What are the likely short-term and long-term effects of this behaviour?

Physical symptoms

Physical symptoms such as headaches, neck and back pain, tiredness, lethargy, abdominal and anxiety-related symptoms may be associated with heartsink. Existing physical health conditions may also be worsened by stress, anxiety and low mood. It is important to identify the impact of these physical reactions upon a GP's daily life.

Environmental factors

Environmental factors also play an important role in the development of heartsink. These include work problems, personal difficulties and life events which cause emotional distress (*Box 19.6*).

Making changes in environmental factors can be an important way of managing negative emotions. For example, choosing to work in a GP practice with supportive or like-minded colleagues or reducing the numbers of hours worked may improve job satisfaction and reduce the frequency of heartsink responses. However, some environmental stresses can be difficult or impossible to change, in which case it is useful to develop more effective coping strategies to manage these difficulties.

Box 19.6

Questions to explore relevant environmental problems

- Are you satisfied with your job? What are the major difficulties?
- Do you have enough support at work and at home?
- Are you maintaining a healthy work/life balance? Do you participate in enjoyable activities outside work?
- Do you have a 'healthy lifestyle' (regular exercise, healthy eating habits, etc.)?
- Are there problems with important personal relationships (family, friends)?
- Are there demands at home (e.g. looking after children or family members)?
- Are there other difficulties (e.g. financial problems, problems with home environment, ill-health, etc.)?
- Have you experienced, or are you about to experience any major life changes?

Case Example 19.1: Using the CBM in heartsink responses

Dr T arrives for a busy morning surgery. When she looks at her list of patients, she notices that Elizabeth is booked in for an appointment at 10 a.m. Elizabeth is 50 years old and presents regularly to the surgery with multiple, changing symptoms. She has been investigated many times, but has never been found to have any serious, organic disease. She is anxious and talkative and Dr T finds it difficult to know how to help her.

As soon as Dr T sees that Elizabeth is on her list, she experiences a heartsink response with the following thoughts, feelings and behaviours:

Thoughts	Feelings
"Oh no, it's Elizabeth! She will make me late for the rest of the surgery." "What does she want this time? There's nothing wrong with her! Seeing her is just wasting my time." "But what if there is really something wrong this time? I could make a major mistake and she would sue me."	Low, anxious and stressed Irritable and angry

Behaviour	Physical symptoms
Distracted and preoccupied by worries about seeing Elizabeth	Headaches
When Elizabeth comes in, tries to rush through the consultation: not listening well, poor eye contact, less empathic than usual	Neck pain
Quick to make a referral / do a test when she complains of a new symptom	Feels exhausted
Environmental factors / triggers	
Difficulties juggling work and child-care arrangements	
In process of trying to sell house; financial difficulties with current mortgage arrangements	

Making changes in heartsink responses

Evaluating thoughts and reframing unhelpful thinking

Once we have discovered the underlying thoughts and beliefs associated with our heartsink reactions, the next stage is to *evaluate* them, in order to identify and reframe any unhelpful or negative automatic thoughts and thinking styles (*Box 19.7*).

Box 19.7	**Checklist for evaluating unhelpful thoughts or beliefs**

- What is the evidence for this thought / belief? Is there any evidence against it?
- Is this an example of an 'unhelpful thinking style'?
- Is it logical or realistic? Is it fair? Is there another way to view the situation?
- Is it helping me to do my job?
- What are the pros and cons of thinking this way?
- What advice would I give to someone else in this situation?
- What is another way to view this situation that takes all of this new evidence into account?

Case Example 19.1: Continued: using the CBM in heartsink responses

Returning to Dr T's feelings of heartsink associated with seeing her patient, Elizabeth, it is helpful to choose the most powerful or distressing 'hot' thought, which can be considered in more depth.

"Oh no, it's Elizabeth! She will make me late for the rest of the surgery.
What does she want this time?
There's nothing wrong with her! Seeing her is just wasting my time.
But what if there is really something wrong this time? I could make a major mistake and she would sue me."

It is possible to test out and evaluate the 'hot' thoughts:

Thought being tested: *"There's nothing wrong with her! Seeing her is just wasting my time."* Feelings associated with this thought: anger, frustration	
What is the evidence for this thought / belief?	*"She doesn't have any evidence of a serious underlying medical condition."* *"She comes in every one to two weeks."* *"The surgery is very busy and short of appointments."*
Is there any evidence against it?	*"She is suffering from really distressing pain and anxiety about her symptoms."* *"Working in primary care means offering support to a variety of patients and problems, not just physical disorders."*
Is this belief an 'unhelpful thinking style'?	All-or-nothing thinking
What are the pros and cons of thinking this way?	Pros: *"important to keep appointments free for other patients who may need them."* Cons: *"makes me feel frustrated; doesn't stop her coming in."*
Is it logical or realistic? Is it fair? Is there another way to view the situation?	*"She is experiencing genuine physical symptoms which she is terrified of. Trying to understand her perspective may help me to feel less frustrated."*
Is it helping me to do my job?	*"Getting annoyed doesn't help me deal with her effectively."*
What advice would I give to someone else in this situation?	*"Take a deep breath and calm down. Take time to get to know the patient and find out what she is most worried about. Plan appointments in advance and be clear about time restrictions."*

What is another way to view this situation that takes all of this new evidence into account?	"Whether I like it or not, seeing patients like Elizabeth is part of my role. Getting angry doesn't help. Building a relationship with her might help reduce her attendances at the surgery."

The following table includes some more alternative, balanced thoughts and perspectives for common negative thoughts in heartsink:

Thought	Unhelpful thinking style	More helpful/balanced alternative thoughts
"I should be able to help this patient otherwise I'm not a good doctor."	Black and white thinking Ignoring the positives	"There is lots of evidence that I am a 'good enough' doctor. No one can be perfect! I have good relationships with many patients and with colleagues. It is not possible to 'cure' everyone – that doesn't mean I am a bad doctor."
"There is nothing I can do to help this woman."	Black and white thinking	"I may not be able to cure this woman's symptoms but I may be able to help her learn to cope better with them. At the very least I can offer empathy and support."
"I could make a major mistake and she would sue me!"	'What if...?' statements Catastrophic thinking	"It is possible that this patient does have something genuinely wrong. However, worrying about it does not help me find out. No one can be 100% certain – I just have to make the best clinical judgement I can."
"The patient blames me for not being able to cure her."	Mind-reading Taking excessive personal responsibility	"She does feel angry and frustrated but she doesn't necessarily think it is my fault. She knows I am trying hard to help her. If she didn't think I could help, she probably wouldn't come back to see me!"

Helpful thoughts and attitudes

Certain beliefs, attitudes and thinking styles can *protect* clinicians from heartsink responses. These are summarised in *Box 19.8*.

Being 'good enough'

It is important for GPs to apply patience and tolerance to themselves as well as others. Being 'good enough' is a key concept for building self-esteem and is highly applicable for many medical practitioners, who often hold perfectionist beliefs and have great difficulty coping with perceived 'failure'.

> "I used to be a real perfectionist and was very hard on myself if even minor problems occurred. I would feel really upset and annoyed with myself if I believed a patient thought badly of me in some way. Now I try to keep a more balanced perspective and remember that I have good relationships with

Box 19.8	**Cognitive factors for managing heartsink reactions**

- Thinking rationally; looking at the bigger picture
- Increased tolerance and patience (acceptance of imperfection in self and others)
- Being able to manage uncertainty
- Learning to make compromises when appropriate
- Being flexible enough to change and learn from patients
- Maintaining a sense of humour (requires a flexible approach to the situation)
- Accepting that we cannot always like or be liked by everyone
- Focusing on long-term as well as short-term goals (e.g. building long-term relationships with patients)

most patients, but it is not possible to do everything for everybody. This helps me cope when things run less smoothly."

Looking at the bigger picture: putting heartsink into perspective

It is often helpful to try to put problems into perspective, by considering whether the situation is really as bad as it seems or whether, in fact, things might be a lot worse!

Case Example 19.2: Putting heartsink experiences into context

Dr B has become increasingly frustrated with one of his patients, Roger. Roger is 82 and suffers from osteoarthritis of the knees which causes him pain and limits his ability to walk. He is also hypertensive and overweight. He frequently attends the surgery but rarely listens to Dr B's advice. Roger says that he can't lose weight and complains of side-effects to most prescribed medication.

Whenever Dr B notices that Roger is on his list, he begins to feel agitated and thinks, *"This man is impossible to help. He doesn't listen to anything I say."* This makes him irritable with Roger and has worsened their relationship.

To try to get some perspective on his difficulties with Roger, Dr B tries a humorous exercise where he imagines the worst possible behaviour that Roger might display in a consultation. For example, Roger might:

- physically attack Dr B or the reception staff
- throw Dr B's computer screen out of the window
- urinate onto Dr B's clothes while being examined

- throw his medication at other patients in the waiting room
- vomit into Dr B's desk drawer whilst the doctor is out of the room

This exercise helped Dr B see Roger with more perspective – Roger is a difficult character to deal with, but his behaviour could be far worse! It is also helpful for Dr B to look at his *own* underlying thoughts and beliefs which may account for his difficulty tolerating Roger's behaviour, such as: "*If patients don't follow my advice it means that they don't respect me.*" This belief can be tested out and evaluated using the checklist for evaluating unhelpful thoughts or beliefs (Box 19.7).

Managing uncertainty

Learning to manage uncertainty is an essential skill for all health professionals. This includes developing and maintaining clinical knowledge and expertise, to ensure that we are competent medical practitioners. However, many *highly competent* GPs still struggle to cope with uncertainty in consultations.

Managing uncertainty involves accepting that we can *never* be 100% certain of anything in life. Good clinical care involves managing *probabilities* rather than certainties and involves making an accurate assessment of the situation. This includes assessing the likelihood of particular risks and behaving accordingly.

> "I used to find it really difficult to cope with uncertainty. I would wake up in the night thinking about a particular patient or wondering whether I missed something. Finally I realised that I can't control everything. I can do my best, but it is impossible to be 100% certain that nothing will ever go wrong. Worrying about these patients at night makes it harder for me to work effectively because I'm tired and stressed out."

> "Of course one day something could go wrong, but that is true for any GP. It is better to deal with this when it actually happens. By continually worrying, I am living through the worst possibilities even before anything bad happens."

From *theory* to *practice*…

Do you hold any beliefs which might make it difficult to cope with uncertainty? Use an example of a concrete, specific situation that you found difficult in order to clearly identify these thoughts.

What is helpful about your belief? Is it also unhelpful in any way? Try re-evaluating and reframing the belief to be more realistic and helpful.

Changing behaviour in heartsink

Changing unhelpful behaviour is an important way of breaking vicious cycles and making positive changes in heartsink situations (*Box 19.9*). Remember, it is not necessary to *feel better* before we *behave* in a more helpful way.

Strategies for changing behaviour

- Make behavioural changes *despite* negative thoughts or feelings
  "What is a more helpful way to behave in this situation? Can I behave like this even if I still experience negative thoughts or feelings?"

- Behave 'as if…'
  "How would I like to feel in this situation? How would I behave differently if I felt that way? Is it possible to behave like this anyway?"

- Modelling others
  "Do I know anyone else who might behave differently in this situation? What would they do? Is it possible for me to try this?"

Using the CBM for teaching, training and mentoring

The CBM approach can be used as an individual self-reflective exercise or used with a trainer, mentor or other colleague. The approach can be applied to understanding heartsink reactions to particular patients, as well as other situations, including work-related stresses and difficulties with colleagues.

Tips for using the CBM with colleagues:

1. **Don't assume you 'know how they feel' (use cognitive empathy)**
    As the mentor or trainer, if you have had a similar experience, you must avoid the temptation of assuming that you know how the 'learner' thinks or feels. Their reaction may be similar in some ways to your own, but is also likely to differ in other ways. Be genuinely interested in discovering the key thoughts, feelings and behaviour that comprise their individual reaction to the problem.

2. **Don't focus purely on the clinical details**
    It can be easy to slip into a clinical discussion about the management of a particular condition, when the learner would benefit more from an exploration of why they found this patient so challenging, by discussing their thoughts and behaviours in that situation.

3. **Write down key information**
   Use a blank CBM chart to write down the key information about thoughts, feelings and behaviours. This helps the learner to distance themselves from the problem and encourages a more flexible view of the situation.

4. **Use specific and concrete examples**
   Ask for specific, recent examples of situations when the learner experienced a difficult situation. Find out exactly what the reaction consisted of and which thoughts underpinned it.

5. **Use collaboration and guided discovery**
   Use the four stages of guided discovery (*Box 19.10*) to encourage the learner to take responsibility for understanding their difficulties and finding appropriate, workable solutions. It is particularly important to hand over responsibility for learning from the discussion (see *Chapter 5* for further details about guided discovery).

Box 19.10

Using guided discovery in teaching and training

1. **Ask informational questions:** use open questions which focus on specific areas of the problem:
   "Give me an example of a situation when you felt this way…"
   "What was going through your mind at that point…?"

2. **Empathic listening and reflection:** listen carefully and express empathic statements if the learner describes any unpleasant or distressing thoughts and feelings:
   "Hmmm – that sounds like it was quite difficult for you…?"

3. **Summarising:** reflect back information as a summary, which encourages the learner to consider the problem from a new perspective:
   "So, this is a patient who behaved in an aggressive way. You started to feel tense because you were thinking, 'he doesn't respect me'. You reacted by becoming defensive and refusing to do what he asked."

4. **'Synthesising' questions:** encourage the learner to make sense of problems themselves:
   "How could you take things forwards…?"
   "Can you see any other way to approach this situation…?"
   "What might you say to a colleague or friend in the same situation…?"

Case Example 19.3: Using the CBM for training and teaching

The following dialogue demonstrates how a GP trainer might use the CBM to discuss a difficult patient with a registrar.

Trainer	Could you start by giving me a brief summary of the patient…?
Registrar	This is a 38 year old woman, who has come in several times with headaches. She has a stressful job in banking. The headaches are classic tension-type pain and she is otherwise well. But she comes in with all kinds of downloads from the internet about headaches and asking for a referral to a neurologist. She can be quite aggressive and demanding in her manner.
Trainer	OK, can you think of a recent time when you saw her?
Registrar	Yes, I saw her two days ago.
Trainer	I'd like us to work through a CBM chart to try to understand your reaction a bit better. At what point did you notice any negative feelings?
Registrar	As soon as I saw she was on my list.
Trainer	How did you feel at that point?
Registrar	I felt tense and fed up.
Trainer	Let's write that down. What was going through your mind that made you feel tense?
Registrar	I was thinking, "*It's going to be another difficult consultation. She will come in and make more demands.*"
Trainer	What is the most difficult part about that? What does it mean to you if she does come in and make demands?
Registrar	I suppose it means that she doesn't respect me as a doctor. She just sees me as a 'tool' to get what she wants.
Trainer	And what would be the worst bit about that? What would that mean about you?
Registrar	That my role is not important – or maybe that I am not important.
Trainer	And how does that make you feel?
Registrar	I suppose I feel a bit hurt, actually.
Trainer	Yes, that makes sense. What you have said so far is that when you were about to see this lady, you started to think: "*It's going to be another difficult consultation. She will come in and make more demands. She doesn't respect me as a doctor. She sees me as a 'tool' to use to get what she wants. And that means that my role is – or I am – not important.*" And those thoughts make you feel a bit hurt. Is that right?
Registrar	Yes, that's right.
Trainer	And do you behave differently with her to any other patients?

Registrar	I think I am more defensive and I listen less to her point of view. I find myself in confrontation with her more than other patients.
Trainer	How do you respond to her demands?
Registrar	I usually comply with them in the end. I did refer her to the neurologist but I felt really annoyed about it.
Trainer	Let's add that to the chart. What made you feel annoyed?
Registrar	I felt I should stand my ground. Giving in to her means that I am letting her get away with making demands and, sort of, pushing me around.
Trainer	Do you have any physical reaction to seeing her?
Registrar	I always feel quite tense and I sometimes get a headache myself.
Trainer	I see. Is there anything else going on at the moment which might affect all this?
Registrar	Well, I am quite busy at the moment, trying to revise for my exams, and also trying to practise my consultation skills, which puts me under extra pressure to consult really well.
Trainer	I see. Well, perhaps you could take a look at everything we have written down. Tell me, what do you make of all this ...?
Registrar	I think maybe I am feeling worse than I need to about how she sees me. She can't think too badly of me or she wouldn't come and see me at all. And I can also see how my being defensive and listening less will make things worse.
Trainer	Yes, that's true. Now, what might be your next steps....?

Key learning points

Summary of the CBM for GP heartsink reactions:

Thoughts and beliefs	Feelings
Critical (of self and others) or intolerant beliefs, perfectionism	Underlying emotional problems (e.g. depression or anxiety)
Unable to cope with uncertainty	Anxiety and worry
Over-dependence on praise, needing to be liked	Stress, frustration, irritability
Defensiveness, difficulty coping with criticism	

Behaviour	Physical symptoms
Deterioration in interpersonal and clinical skills when tense and stressed	Tension and stress-related physical symptoms
Reassurance-seeking or avoidance	
Difficulty making decisions	
Reduced self-care	
Poor work–life balance: lack of enjoyable activities	

Environment and background
Complex or other patients perceived to be 'challenging' (e.g. frequent attendances)
Less experienced doctors, lacking training in communication skills
Difficulties in the workplace: low job satisfaction, high perceived workload
Personal worries and life events

- Heartsink reactions are unpleasant negative feelings which arise in health professionals when faced by particular patients or situations.
- GPs who are more likely to experience heartsink include those with low job satisfaction or who need to develop their communication skills. So, noticing a lot of heartsink reactions may sometimes indicate that you need to undertake some training or make changes in other areas of your life or work.
- Heartsink can also be a symptom of burnout or emotional disorders such as depression and anxiety. Make sure you visit your own GP if you suspect this may be the case.
- To change heartsink reactions, GPs must take responsibility for their own thoughts and feelings and avoid blaming or labelling patients.

Key strategies in managing heartsink include:
- Improve your understanding and communication skills for working with patient groups that you find particularly challenging such as health anxiety and MUS (see *Chapter 15*).
- Keep things in perspective – ask yourself how important will this be in five years?
- Don't be a perfectionist – focus on being 'good enough' and remember that you can't be liked by everyone.
- Work on your ability to tolerate uncertainty. This can be very challenging for many GPs. Remember that we can never be 100% certain of anything in life.

- Try to build your patience, tolerance and empathy for others.
- Keep a sense of humour!
- When under pressure, focus on behaving 'as if' you felt better. Behavioural changes are the most effective way to break vicious cycles in heartsink reactions.

References and further reading

References

American Psychiatric Association (1994) *Diagnostic and Statistical Manual of Mental Disorders,* 4th edn. American Psychiatric Association, Washington, DC.

Babyak M, Blumenthal JA, Herman S, *et al.* (2000) Exercise treatment for major depression: maintenance of therapeutic benefit at 10 months. *Psychosomatic Medicine* **62**: 633–8.

Barry CA, Bradley C, Britten N, *et al.* (2000) Patients' unvoiced agendas in general practice consultations: qualitative study. *British Medical Journal* **320**: 1246–50.

Barsky A, Ahern, D (2004) Cognitive behavior therapy for hypochondriasis: randomized controlled trial. *Journal of the American Medical Association* **291**: 1464–70.

Bass C, Murphy M (1995) Somatoform and personality disorders: syndromal comorbidity and overlapping developmental pathways. *Journal of Psychosomatic Research* **39**: 403–27.

Beck AT, Emery G, Greenberg RL (1985) *Anxiety Disorders and Phobias: a Cognitive Perspective.* Basic Books, New York.

Beck AT, Rush AJ, Shaw BF, Emery G (1979) *Cognitive Therapy of Depression.* Guilford Press, New York.

Breivik H, Collett B, Ventafridda V, Cohen R, Gallacher D (2006) Survey of chronic pain in Europe: prevalence, impact on daily life, and treatment. *European Journal of Pain* **10**: 287–333.

Burns D, Nolen-Hoeksema S (1991) Coping styles, homework compliance, and the effectiveness of cognitive-behavioral therapy. *Journal of Consulting and Clinical Psychology* **59**: 305–11.

Butler CC, Evans M (1999) The heartsink patient revisited. *British Journal of General Practice* **49**: 230–3.

Clark DM (1986) A cognitive model of panic. *Behaviour Research and Therapy* **24**: 461–70.

Craig TK, Boardman AP (1997) ABC of mental health: common mental health problems in primary care. *British Medical Journal* **314**: 1609–13.

Department of Health (2001) *Treatment Choice in Psychological Therapies and Counselling.* Department of Health, London.

Department of Health (2008) *Improving Access to Psychological Therapies: Long-term conditions positive practice guide.* Department of Health, London.

Dimidjian S, Hollon SD, Dobson KS, *et al.* (2006) Randomized trial of behavioral activation, cognitive therapy, and anti-depressant medication in the acute treatment of adults with major depression. *Journal of Consulting and Clinical Psychology* **74**: 658–70.

Escobar JI, Gara MA, Diaz-Martinez AM, *et al.* (2007) Effectiveness of a time-limited cognitive behavior therapy-type intervention among primary care patients with medically unexplained symptoms. *Annals of Family Medicine* **5**: 328–35.

Greenberger D, Padesky CA (1995a) *Mind over Mood.* Guilford Press, New York.

Greenberger D, Padesky CA (1995b) *Clinician's Guide to Mind over Mood.* Guilford Press, New York.

Harris R (2006) Embracing your demons: an overview of acceptance and commitment therapy. *Psychotherapy in Australia* **12**(4): 2–7.

Hasenbring MI, Rusu AC, Turk DC (2012) From acute to chronic back pain: risk factors, mechanisms, and clinical implications. *Oxford Medicine Online.* Available at: http://oxfordmedicine.com/view/10.1093/med/9780199558902.001.0001/med-9780199558902 (last accessed 9 May 2013)

Hayes SC, Strosahl KD, Wilson KG (1999) *Acceptance and Commitment Therapy: An experiential approach to behavior change.* Guilford Press, New York.

Horvath AO, Symonds BD (1991) Relation between working alliance and outcome in psychotherapy: a meta-analysis. *Journal of Counseling Psychology* **38**: 139–49.

Kabat-Zinn J (1990) *Full Catastrophe Living: Using the Wisdom of Your Mind and Body to Face Stress, Pain and Illness.* Delta, New York.

Kabat-Zinn J, Lipworth L, Burney R, Sellers W (1986) Four year follow-up of a meditation-based program for the self-regulation of chronic pain: treatment outcomes and compliance. *Clinical Journal of Pain* **2**: 159–73.

Kabat-Zinn J, Massio AO, Kristeller J, *et al.* (1992) Effectiveness of a meditation-based stress reduction program in the treatment of anxiety disorders. *American Journal of Psychiatry* **149**: 936–43.

Kabat-Zinn J, Wheeler E, Light T, *et al.* (1998) Influence of a mindfulness meditation-based stress reduction intervention on rates of skin clearing in patients with moderate to severe psoriasis undergoing phototherapy (UVB) and phytochemotherapy (PUVA). *Psychosomatic Medicine* **60**: 625–32.

Katon W, Schulberg H (1992) Epidemiology of depression in primary care. *General Hospital Psychiatry* **14**: 237–47.

Kennedy TM, Jones R, Darnley S, *et al.* (2005) Cognitive behavioural therapy in addition to antispasmodic therapy for irritable bowel syndrome in primary care: randomised controlled trial. *British Medical Journal* **331**: 435–7.

Kennerley H (1997) *Overcoming Anxiety.* Constable and Robinson, London.

Kessler RC, McGonagle KA, Zhao S, *et al.* (1994) Lifetime and 12-month prevalence of DSM-IIIR psychiatric disorders in the United States: results of the national comorbidity survey. *Archives of General Psychiatry* **51**: 8–19.

Kroenke K (2007) Efficacy of treatment for somatoform disorders: a review of randomized controlled trials. *Psychosomatic Medicine* **69**: 881–8.

Mathers N, Jones N, Hannay D (1995) Heartsink patients: a study of their general practitioners. *British Journal of General Practice* **45**: 293–6.

Melzack R, Wall PD (1965) Pain mechanisms: a new theory. *Science* **150**: 971–9.

Mendell LM, Wall PD (1965) Responses of single dorsal cells to peripheral cutaneous unmyelinated fibers. *Nature* **206**: 97–9.

Mumford DB, Devereux TA, Maddy PJ, *et al.* (1991) Factors leading to the reporting of 'functional' somatic symptoms by general practitioners. *British Journal of General Practice* **41**: 454–8.

National Institute for Health and Clinical Excellence (NICE) (2008) Commissioning Guide: *Cognitive Behavioural Therapy for the management of common mental health problems.* NICE, London.

National Institute for Health and Clinical Excellence (NICE) (2009a) CG22: *Depression: management of depression in primary and secondary care.* NICE, London.

National Institute for Health and Clinical Excellence (NICE) (2009b) CG91: *Depression in adults with a chronic physical health problem: treatment and management.* NICE, London.

National Institute for Health and Clinical Excellence (NICE) (2011) CG113: *Generalised anxiety disorder and panic disorder (with or without agoraphobia) in adults.* NICE, London.

Nezu AM, Nezu CM (1989) *Problem-solving Therapy for Depression: Theory, research and clinical guidelines.* Wiley, New York.

Orlinsky D, Grawe K, Parks B (1994) Process and outcome in psychotherapy. In: *Handbook of Psychotherapy and Behavior Change* (Bergin A, Garfield S, Eds). Wiley: New York.

Padesky CA (1993) Schema as self-prejudice. *International Cognitive Therapy Newsletter* **5/6**: 16–7.

Padesky CA (2003) *Guided Discovery: Leading and Following (audiotape).* Centre for Cognitive Therapy, California.

Padesky CA, Mooney KA (1990) Clinical tip: presenting the cognitive model to clients. *International Cognitive Therapy Newsletter* **6**: 13–4.

Paykel ES, Scott J, Teasdale JD, et al. (1999) Prevention of relapse in residual depression by cognitive therapy: a controlled trial. *Archives of General Psychiatry* **56**: 829–35.

Peveler R, Kilkenny L, Kinmonth AL (1997) Medically unexplained physical symptoms in primary care: a comparison. *Journal of Psychosomatic Research* **42**: 245–52.

Rollnick S, Miller WR, Butler C (2008) *Motivational Interviewing in Health Care: helping patients change behavior.* Guilford Press, London.

Roth A, Fonagy P (2005) *What Works for whom? 2nd Edn.* Guilford Press: New York.

Roth A, Pilling S (2007) *The Competences Required to Deliver Effective Cognitive and Behavioural Therapy for People with Depression and with Anxiety Disorders.* Department of Health: London.

Rubak S, Sandbaek A, Lauritzen T, Christensen B (2005) Motivational interviewing: a systematic review and meta-analysis. *British Journal of General Practice* **55**: 305–12.

Safran J, Segal Z (1990) *Interpersonal Processes in Cognitive Therapy.* Basic Books, New York.

Safran J, Segal Z, Vallis, T, Shaw B, Samstag L (1993) Assessing patient suitability for short-term cognitive therapy with an interpersonal focus. *Cognitive Therapy & Research,* **17**: 23–8.

Salmon P, Peters S, Stanley I (1999) Patients' perceptions of medical explanations for somatisation disorders: qualitative analysis. *British Medical Journal* **318**: 372–6.

Scott C, Tacchi MJ, Jones R, Scott J (1997) Acute and one-year outcome of a RCT of brief cognitive therapy for major depressive disorder in primary care. *British Journal of Psychiatry* **171**: 131–4.

Segal ZV, Williams JMG, Teasdale JD (2001) *Mindfulness-based Cognitive Therapy for Depression. A new approach to preventing relapse.* Guilford Press, New York.

Speckens AE, Van Hemert AM, Spinhoven P, et al. (1995) Cognitive behavioural therapy for medically unexplained physical symptoms: a randomised controlled trial. *British Medical Journal* **311**: 1328–32.

Steinmetz D, Tabenkin H (2001) The 'difficult patient' as perceived by family physicians. *Family Practice* **18**: 495–500.

Waddell G, Burton A, Kendall NO (2008) *Vocational Rehabilitation: what works, for whom, and when?* The Stationery Office, London.

Warwick H, Salkovskis P (1989) Hypochondriasis. In: *Cognitive Therapy in Clinical Practice: an Illustrated Casebook* (Scott J, Mark J, Williams G, Beck AT, Eds), pp. 78–102. Routledge, London.

Warwick HM, Clark DM, Cobb AM, Salkovskis PM (1996) A controlled trial of cognitive-behavioural treatment of hypochondriasis. *British Journal of Psychiatry* **169**: 189–95.

Wells A (1997) *Cognitive Therapy of Anxiety Disorders.* Chichester, John Wiley and Sons.

Westbrook D, Kennerley H, Kirk J (2007) *An Introduction to Cognitive Behaviour Therapy: skills and applications.* Sage Publications Ltd, London.

White PD, Goldsmith KA, Johnson AL, et al. (2011) Comparison of adaptive pacing therapy, cognitive behaviour therapy, graded exercise therapy, and specialist medical care for chronic fatigue syndrome (PACE): a randomised trial. *Lancet* **377**: 823–36.

Williams CJ, Garland A (2002) A cognitive-behavioural assessment model for use in everyday clinical practice. *Advances in Psychiatric Treatment* **8**: 172–9.

Further reading

Armstrong D (1996) Construct validity and GPs' perceptions of psychological problems. *Primary Care Psychiatry* **2**: 119–122.

Balint M (1964) *The Doctor, His Patient and The Illness.* Churchill Livingstone, Edinburgh.

Barsky AJ, Wyshak G, Klerman GL, Latham KS (1990) The prevalence of hypochondriasis in medical outpatients. *Social Psychiatry and Psychiatric Epidemiology* **25**: 89–90.

Bass C, May S (2002) ABC of psychological medicine: Chronic multiple functional somatic symptoms. *British Medical Journal* **325**: 323–6.

Beck AT (1976) *Cognitive Therapy and the Emotional Disorders.* International Universities Press, New York.

Beck AT, Weishaar M (1986) Cognitive therapy. In: *Cognitive Behavioural Approaches to Psychotherapy* (Dryden W, Golden W, eds), pp. 61–92. Harper & Row, London.

Beck J (1995) *Cognitive Therapy: Basics and Beyond.* Guilford Press, New York.

Becker MH, Maiman LA (1975) Sociobehavioural determinants of compliance with medical care recommendations. *Medical Care* **13**: 10–24.

Bennett-Levy J, Butler G, Fennell M, et al. (Eds) (2004) *Oxford Guide to Behavioural Experiments in Cognitive Therapy.* Oxford University Press, Oxford.

Berne E (1964) *Games People Play.* Grove Press, New York.

Blackburn IM, James IA, Baker C, *et al.* (2001) The revised cognitive therapy scale (CTS-R): psychometric properties. *Behavioural and Cognitive Psychotherapy* **29**: 431–46.

Bracken P, Thomas P (2001) Post psychiatry: a new direction for mental health. *British Medical Journal* **322**: 724–727.

Britten N, Stevenson FA, Barry CA, Barber N, Bradley CP (2000) Misunderstandings in prescribing decisions in general practice: qualitative study. *British Medical Journal* **320**: 484–8.

Butler C, Pill R, Stott N (1998) Qualitative study of patients' perceptions of doctors' advice to quit smoking: implications for opportunistic health promotion. *British Medical Journal* **316**: 1878–81.

Butler G (1999) *Overcoming Social Anxiety and Shyness.* Constable and Robinson, London.

Churchill R, Khaira M, Gretton V *et al.* (2000) Treating depression in general practice: factors affecting patients' treatment preferences. *British Journal of General Practice* **460**: 905–906.

Crutcher JE, Bass MJ (1980) The difficult patient and the troubled physician. *Journal of Family Practice* **11**: 933–8.

Davidson O, King M, Sharp D, Taylor F (1999) A pilot randomised trial evaluating GP registrar management of major depression following brief training in cognitive-behaviour therapy. *Education in General Practice* **10**: 485–8.

Double D (2002) The limits of psychiatry. *British Medical Journal* **324**: 900–4.

Enright SJ (1997) Cognitive-behaviour therapy – clinical applications. *British Medical Journal* **314**: 1811–1816.

Fennell M (1999) *Overcoming Low Self-esteem.* Constable and Robinson, London.

Fitzpatrick R (1996) Telling patients there is nothing wrong (editorial). *British Medical Journal* **313**: 311–2.

Friedberg R, Fideleo R (1992) Training in-patient staff in cognitive therapy. *Journal of Cognitive Psychotherapy* **6**: 105–12.

Gilbert P (2000) *Overcoming Depression.* Constable and Robinson, London.

Gill D, Hatcher S (2000) Antidepressants for depression in medical illness. *Cochrane Database of Systematic Reviews* **4**: CD0001312.

Goldberg DP, Steele JJ, Smith C, Spivey L (1980) Training family doctors to recognize psychiatric illness with increased accuracy. *Lancet* **2**: 521–3.

Greeven *et al.* (2007) Cognitive behavior therapy and paroxetine in the treatment of hypochondriasis: a randomized controlled trial. *American Journal of Psychiatry* **164**: 91–9.

Hale A (1998) *ABC of Mental Health.* BMJ Books, London.

Hawton K, Salkovskis PM, Kirk J, Clark DM (Eds) (1989) *Cognitive Behaviour Therapy for Psychiatric Problems. A Practical Guide.* Oxford University Press, Oxford.

Hayes, SC, Smith S (2005) *Get Out of Your Mind and Into Your Life: The New Acceptance and Commitment Therapy.* New Harbinger Publications, Oakland, CA.

Hayes SC, Strosahl KD, Wilson KG (2011) Acceptance and Commitment Therapy: The Process and Practice of Mindful Change (2nd ed.). Guilford Press, New York.

Heath I (1999) Commentary: There must be limits to the medicalization of human distress. *British Medical Journal* **318**: 440.

Helman CG (1990) *Culture, Health & Illness.* Butterworth-Heinemann, Oxford.

Hodgson P, Smith P, Brown T, Dowrick C (2005) Stories from frequent attenders: a qualitative study in primary care. *Annals of Family Medicine* **3**: 318–23.

House A, Stark D (2002) ABC of psychological medicine: Anxiety in medical patients. *British Medical Journal* **325**: 207–209.

Jacobson N, Martell CR, Dimidjan S. Behavioral Activation for depression: Returning to contextual roots. *Clinical Psychology: Science and Practice* **8**: 255–270.

Kadam U, Croft P, McLeod J, Hutchinson M (2001) A qualitative study of patients' views on anxiety and depression. *British Journal of General Practice* **466**: 375–380.

Kenardy J (2003) Review: cognitive behaviour therapy and behaviour therapy may be effective for back pain and chronic fatigue syndrome, and antidepressants may be effective for irritable bowel syndrome. *Evidence Based Medicine* **8**: 88.

King M, Davidson O, Taylor F, et al. (2002) Effectiveness of teaching general practitioners skills in brief cognitive behaviour therapy to treat patients with depression: randomised controlled trial. *British Medical Journal* **324**: 927–36.

Kurtz S, Silverman J, Draper J (2004) *Teaching and Learning Communication Skills in Medicine.* Radcliffe Medical Press, Oxford.

Launer J (2002) *Narrative-based Primary Care: a Practical Guide.* Radcliffe Medical Press, Oxford.

Marks JN, Goldberg DP, Hillier VF (1979) Determinants of the ability of general practitioners to detect psychiatric illness. *Psychological Medicine* **9**: 337–54.

Mathers N, Gask L (1995) Surviving the 'heartsink' experience. *Family Practice* **12**: 176–83.

Mayou R, Farmer A (2002) Functional somatic symptoms and syndromes. *British Medical Journal* **325**: 265–8.

McCrone P, Sharpe M, Chalder T, Knapp M, Johnson AL, et al. (2011) Adaptive Pacing, Cognitive Behaviour Therapy, Graded Exercise, and Specialist Medical Care for Chronic Fatigue Syndrome: A Cost-Effectiveness Analysis. *Lancet* **377**: 823–36.

McDonald IG, Daly J, Jelinek JM, Panetta F, Gutman JM (1996) Opening Pandora's box: the unpredictability of reassurance by a normal test result. *British Medical Journal* **313**: 329–32.

Mercer SW, Reilly D, Watt GC (2002) The importance of empathy in the enablement of patients attending the Glasgow Homoeopathic Hospital. *British Journal of General Practice* **52**: 901–5.

Michie S, Rumsey N, Fussell A, Hardeman W, Johnston MM, Newman S, Yardley L (2006) *Improving Health: Changing Behaviour* NHS Health Trainer Handbook. Department of Health, London.

Middleton H, Shaw I (2000) Distinguishing mental illness in primary care (editorial). *British Medical Journal* **320**: 1420.

Miller WR, Rollnick S (2002) Motivational interviewing: preparing people for change (2nd ed Guilford Press, New York.

Moral RR, Alamo MM, Jurado AM, Perula de Torres L (2001) Effectiveness of a learner-centred training programme for primary care physicians in using a patient-centred consultation style. *Family Practice* **18**(1): 60–63.

Murray CJ, Lopez AD (1997) Alternative projections of mortality and disability by cause 1990–2020: global burden of disease study. *Lancet* **349**: 1498–504.

Murray CJ, Lopez AD (1997) Regional patterns of disability-free life expectancy and disability adjusted life expectancy: global burden of disease study. *Lancet* **349**: 1347–52.

Mynors-Wallis L (1996) Problem-solving treatment: evidence for effectiveness and feasibility in primary care. *International Journal of Psychiatry in Medicine* **26**: 249–62.

Mynors-Wallis L (2005) *Problem-Solving Treatment for Anxiety and Depression: A Practical Guide.* Oxford University Press, Oxford.

Mynors-Wallis LM, Gath DH, Day A, Baker F (1995) RCT comparing problem solving treatment with amitriptyline and placebo for major depression in primary care. *British Medical Journal* **310**: 441–5.

National Collaborating Centre for Mental Health (2004) *Eating Disorders: Core Interventions in the Treatment and Management of Anorexia Nervosa, Bulimia Nervosa and Related Eating Disorders.* The British Psychological Society and the Royal College of Psychiatrists, Leicester and London.

National Institute for Clinical Excellence (NICE) (2004) CG22: *Depression: Management of Depression in Primary and Secondary Care.* NICE, London.

National Institute for Clinical Excellence (NICE) (2004) CG23: *Anxiety: Management of Anxiety in Primary, Secondary and Community Care.* NICE, London.

National Institute for Clinical Excellence (NICE) (2005) CG26: *Post-traumatic stress disorder (PTSD).* NICE, London.

National Institute for Clinical Excellence (NICE) (2005) CG31: *Obsessive Compulsive Disorder.* NICE, London.

National Institute for Health and Clinical Excellence (NICE) (2007) CG53: *Chronic fatigue syndrome/myalgic encephalomyelitis (or encephalopathy): diagnosis and management of CFS/ME in adults and children.* NICE, London.

Neenan M, Dryden W (2002) *Cognitive Behaviour Therapy: An A-Z of Persuasive Arguments.* Whurr Publishers, London.

Neighbour R (1987) *The Inner Consultation.* Churchill Livingstone, Edinburgh.

Neighbour R (1996) *The Inner Apprentice.* Petroc Press, Newbury.

O'Dowd TC (1988) Five years of heartsink patients in general practice. *British Medical Journal* **297**: 528–32.

Pendleton D, Schofield T, Tate P, Havelock P (2002) *The Consultation: An Approach to Learning and Teaching.* Oxford University Press, Oxford.

Persons, J (1989) *Cognitive Therapy in Practice. A Case Formulation Approach.* W.W. Norton, New York.

Peveler R, Carson A, Rodin G (2002) ABC of psychological medicine: Depression in medical patients. *British Medical Journal* **325**: 149–152.

Pollock K, Grime J (2002) Patients' perceptions of entitlement to time in general practice consultations for depression: a qualitative study. *British Medical Journal* **325**: 687–92.

Raine R, Haines A, Sensky T, Hutchings A, Larkin K, Black N (2002) Systematic review of mental health interventions for patients with common somatic symptoms: can research evidence from secondary care be extrapolated to primary care? *British Medical Journal* **325**: 1082.

Rimes KA, Chalder T (2010) The Beliefs about Emotions Scale: validity, reliability and sensitivity to change. *Psychosom Res.* **68**(3): 285–92.

Ring A, Dowrick C, Humphris G, Salmon P (2004) Do patients with unexplained physical symptoms pressurize general practitioners for somatic treatment? A qualitative study. *British Medical Journal* **328**: 1319–20.

Ring A, Dowrick CF, Humphris GM, Davies J, Salmon P (2005) The somatizing effect of clinical consultation: what patients and doctors say and do not say when patients present medically unexplained physical symptoms. *Social Science Medicine* **61**: 1505–15.

Rollnick S, Butler CC, Kinnersley P, Gregory J, Mash B (2010) Motivational interviewing. *British Medical Journal* **340**: 1900.

Sage N, Sowden M, Chorlton E, Edeleanu A (2008) *CBT for Chronic Illness and Palliative Care: a workbook and toolkit.* John Wiley & Sons Ltd, Chichester.

Salkovskis P, Bass C (1997) Hypochondriasis. In: *Science and Practice of Cognitive Behaviour Therapy* (Clark D, Fairburn C, eds). Oxford University Press, Oxford.

Salkovskis P, Clark D (1993) Panic disorder and hypochondriasis. *Advances in Behaviour Research and Therapy* **15**: 23–48.

Sanders D (1996) *Counselling for Psychosomatic Problems.* Sage, London.

Say R, Thomson R (2003) The importance of patient preference in treatment decisions – challenges for doctors. *British Medical Journal* **327**: 542–545.

Silverman J, Kurtz S, Draper J (1998) *Skills for Communicating with Patients.* Radcliffe Medical Press, Oxford.

Stopa L, Thorne P (1999) Cognitive-behavioural therapy training: teach the formulation first. *Clinical Psychology Forum* **123**: 20–3.

Teasale JD, Segal Z, Williams JMG, *et al.* (2000) Prevention of relapse/recurrence in major depression by mindfulness-based cognitive therapy. *Journal of Consulting and Clinical Psychology* **68**: 615–23.

Thomas E, Silman AS, Croft PR, *et al.* (1999) Predicting who develops chronic low back pain: a prospective study. *British Medical Journal* **318**: 1662–7.

Thompson C, Kinmonth AL, Stevens L *et al.* (2000) Effects of a clinical-practice guideline and practice-based education on detection and outcome of depression in primary care: Hampshire Depression Project randomised controlled trial. *Lancet* **355**: 185–191.

Van Tulder M, Ostelo R, Vlaeyen J, *et al.* (2000) Behavioural treatment for chronic low back pain. *Cochrane Database of Systematic Reviews* **2**: CD002014.

Ward E, King M, Lloyd M, *et al.* (2000) Randomised controlled trial of non-directive counselling, cognitive-behaviour therapy and usual general practitioner care for patients with depression I: clinical effectiveness. *British Medical Journal* **321**: 1383–8.

Wells KB, Stewart A, Hays RD, *et al.* (1989) The functioning and well-being of depressed patients. Results from the medical outcomes study. *Journal of the American Medical Association* **262**: 914–9.

White C (2001) *Cognitive Behaviour Therapy for Chronic Medical Problems.* John Wiley and Sons, Chichester.

Williams CJ (2001) *Overcoming Depression: A Five Areas Approach.* Arnold, London.

Wills F, Sanders D (1997) *Cognitive Therapy: transforming the image.* Sage, London.

Training for health professionals

British Association of Behavioural and Cognitive Psychotherapies (BABCP)

BABCP (www.babcp.com) is a multidisciplinary interest group for professionals involved in theory and practice of CBT. The website offers a very useful resource which:

- Gives information about CBT training and events throughout the UK
- Contains printable brief patient leaflets
- Provides details of accredited CBT practitioners, searchable by area. Patients can self-refer to private therapists.

10 Minute CBT Training

Dr Lee David runs workshops for GPs and other primary care health professionals on using the '10 minute CBT' approach outlined in this book. For further details on upcoming events or to arrange a training event in your area, e-mail office@10minuteCBT.co.uk or look at www.10minuteCBT.co.uk. The website also contains useful printable CBT leaflets for patients.

10 Minute CBT DVDs

There are three training DVDs which have been developed specifically to demonstrate the 10 Minute CBT techniques and communication skills described in this book. The titles are:

- Mental health
- Physical health and long-term conditions
- Health anxiety and medically unexplained symptoms

All DVDs can be purchased via the 10 Minute CBT website.

Index